I0440022

Good Sleep for Brain Health

Sleep Better Tonight for a Better Memory Tomorrow

M. Chris Wolf, PhD

Author of

Brain Health: Simple Steps to a Better Memory

http://www.amazon.com/Brain-Health-Simple-Better-ebook/dp/B008S9A9I8

Published by:

Memory Loss Facts

1701 Williams Court

Columbus, GA 31904 USA

www.Memory-Loss-Facts.com

Copyright © 2013 by M. Chris Wolf, PhD

M. Chris Wolf, PhD

DISCLAIMER AND LEGAL NOTICES

This eBook is an educational health and fitness related information product.

The information presented within this Book solely and fully represents the views of the author as of the date of publication. Any slight to, or potential misrepresentation of, any person or companies is entirely unintentional. As a result of changing information, conditions or contexts, this author reserves the right to alter content or option with impunity. The information contained within is not intended to provide specific physical or mental health advice, or any other advice whatsoever, for any individual or company and should not be relied upon in that regard.

There may be risks related to participating in activities or using products for people with pre-existing illness, poor health, or mental illness.

As these risks exist, you are not to use these products or participate in activities if you have pre-existing illness, poor health, or mental illness. Should you choose to participate in these risks, you do so of your free will and accord, being made aware and voluntarily participating in these risks. It is suggested to visit a certified medical practitioner before making any changes to your diet or lifestyle.

Author's Notes

Please enjoy my companion website where there are valuable informational pages on memory improvement and updates are available to my readers. You will also find links to my other books and publications related to brain health and memory functioning.

Please Review This Book

I want to ask you a favor ... Could you PLEASE head back over to Amazon. com and **REVIEW** this book?

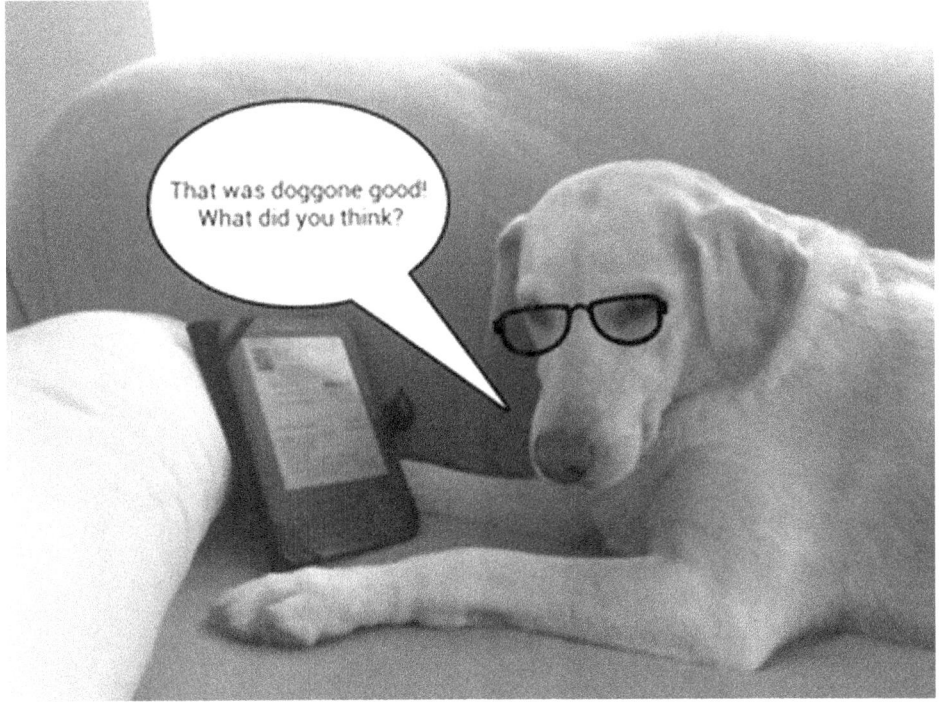

I need your feedback to make the next version better.

Thank you so much!

M. Chris Wolf, PhD

Contents

Introduction

If you are on one of the millions of Americans who will go to bed tonight wondering whether you will be able to sleep, you need to read this book. As you are reading this introduction, millions of people around the globe are struggling with a disturbance of sleep.

Sleep deprivation has been identified as a cause of poor cognitive fitness, memory loss, depression, anxiety, and industrial and traffic accidents. Research has also identified poor sleep quality as a contributing factor to disease states such as diabetes, high blood pressure, and various cancers.

Jonathan (not his real name), a former patient of mine, is a soldier who has survived three deployments to combat. As he walks into his bedroom, he feels anxious and discouraged. He dreads the night because he has an early formation in the morning and cannot sleep. Anticipatory anxiety about frequent, intrusive nightmares keeps him up most nights until he eventually crashes.

Emily has not been sleeping well for months since she and her husband split. She is a single parent and worries that she will not be able to manage on her own. She is usually awake for two to three hours each night, lying in bed before she finally falls asleep. In the morning she often sleeps through her alarm.

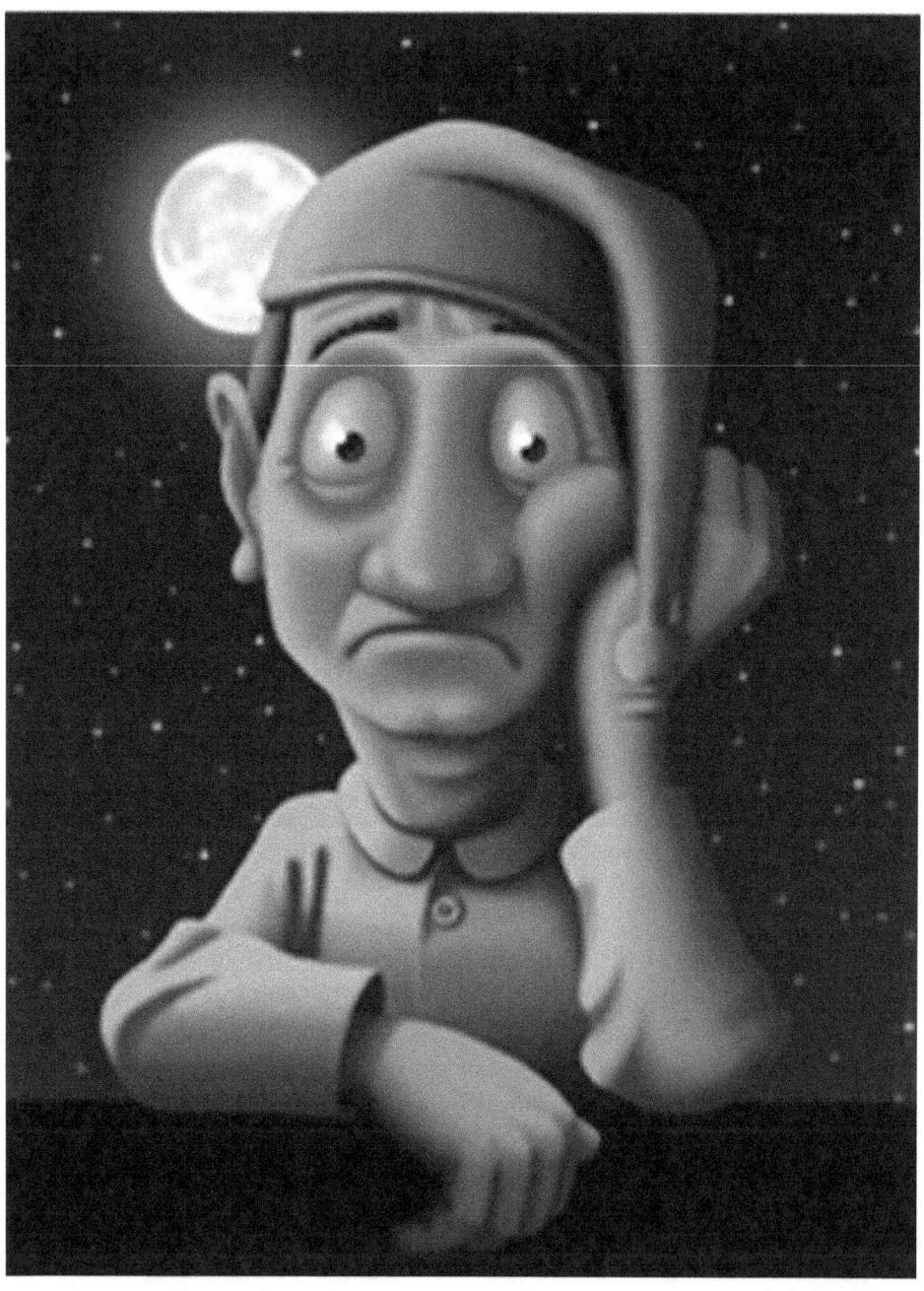

Bob has a two-year-old who has a breathing problem that often emerges at night. He has not slept well since his son, Josh, was diagnosed with the disorder. Most mornings he is so tired he has difficulty getting organized. He now drinks energy drinks to get by, and he sometimes adds one in the afternoon. He worries that his personality has changed.

Louise has not slept well since Richard began developing dementia several years ago. One night she awoke and found him standing in the driveway of their home confused and disoriented. He has taken to wandering, and she worries he will be hurt or even hit by a car.

These people and millions like them around the world have developed a sleep disturbance that haunts them. As the days, weeks, and months go by, they begin to notice changes in their mood, personality, energy level and memory. As previously noted, researchers now know that sleep deprivation can cause a myriad of health and psychological problems ranging from cardiovascular disease to depression.

Methods to enhance sleep and prevent sleep loss and insomnia are well known. The research evidence is now available. While there is sometimes a medical reason for insomnia and poor sleep quality, there are also habit patterns that may be the main culprit.

In this book we will examine how a person's psychological and physical health can be affected by sleep problems. Most importantly, we will give you specific suggestions for improving your sleep, thereby improving your health and well-being.

This book provides a road map for the average person to be able to identify whether professional help is required. Oftentimes, sleep problems can be resolved without a professional.

Once you have identified with which group you are a member, you can move forward to eliminate your sleep deprivation problem now and into the future. Even if you decide that professional help is necessary, this book will provide the guidance you need to communicate more effectively about your sleep problem with a healthcare professional.

According to the Centers for Disease Control (CDC), approximately 50–70 million US adults have sleep disorders of various kinds. The CDC data also indicates that snoring is a major indicator of obstructive sleep apnea (OSA). OSA can be life threatening, and as we will discuss, contributes to poor cardiovascular and brain health. Do you snore?

As previously alluded to, sleep is also increasingly recognized as important to occupational health, with sleep insufficiency linked to motor vehicle crashes, industrial disasters, and medical and other occupational errors.

Did you know that people experiencing sleep deficits are also more likely to suffer from chronic disease such as a diabetes, hypertension, obesity and depression? Cancer, increased death rates, and reduced quality of life and productivity are also all associated with sleep insufficiency. All of these things relate directly or indirectly to brain health and your memory functions.

Over many years, I have worked with many people who have benefited from the methods outlined in this book. Proper sleep hygiene can be learned by almost anyone willing to follow simple steps to a better night's sleep. The best research available in health, behavioral medicine, and neuroscience has been done and is presented for you in this book without the jargon so that you can begin to make changes tonight.

Whether you suffer from a sleep disturbance that is acute and has come on in less than 30 days, or one that is more chronic and has lasted over three months or more, this book is for you.

The vast majority of people who implement this sleep-wise approach sleep better almost immediately. Many make major improvements in their sleep within 30 days. Some people have been able to eliminate prescription and nonprescription drugs in collaboration with their healthcare provider. Do you want to be part of this group? Do you want to learn about how sleep affects your health and especially your memory?

Most importantly, you will be able to develop an individual plan of care to help you resolve the problem. Many people find that they can improve their sleep quickly, while some others will take a little more time. Everybody, though, can improve their sleep, if only a little.

Each night you spend with disrupted sleep increases the probability that you will develop the negative effects of sleep deprivation noted earlier. You can improve your physical, brain, and mental health by sleeping better tonight. You can increase the depth and quality of your sleep in the coming days and months.

Finally, if you decide that you need professional assistance, you will have a better idea of what is happening and how and what to communicate to your health care provider.

Turn to Chapter One and invest six minutes to learn how you can improve your sleep tonight for a better brain and physical health tomorrow. Let's get started.

M. Chris Wolf, PhD

Why Is Poor Sleep a Concern for Your Brain?

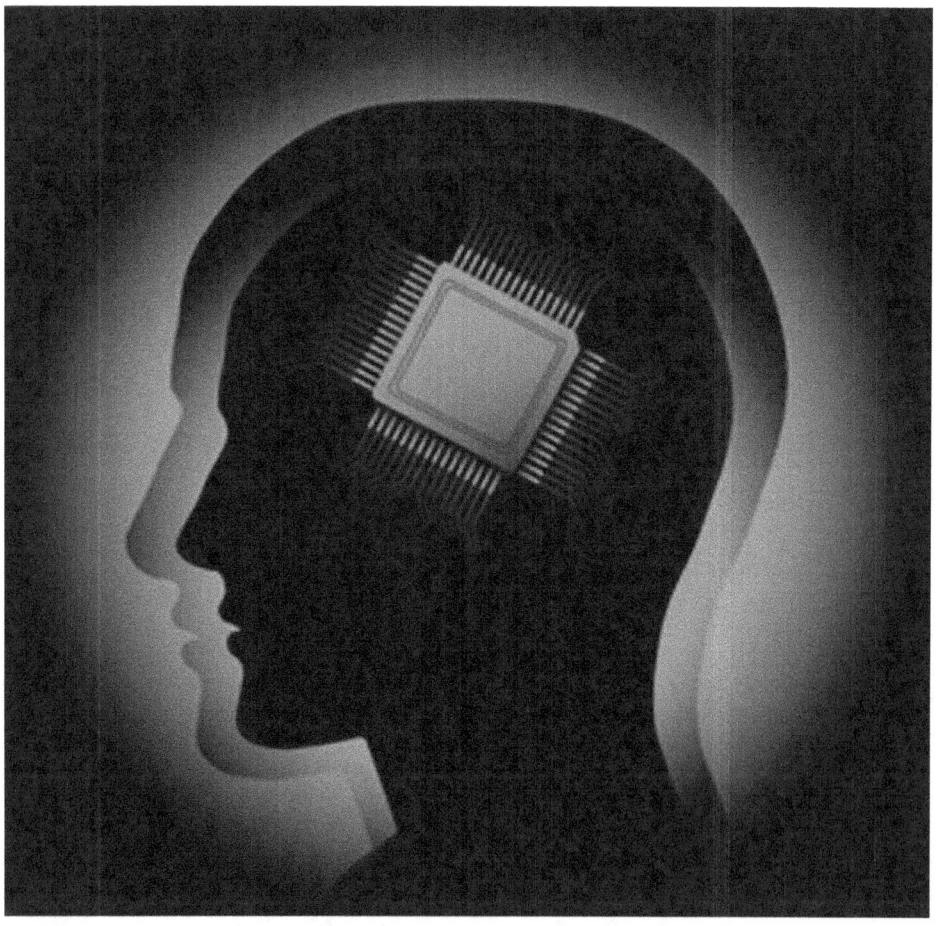

Sleep deprived people don't perform well. Insomnia has been identified as a major risk factor for the development of new emotional problems. (1) People are sleeping less every year. According to the National Sleep Foundation, 63 percent of Americans report that they do not meet their need for sleep during a typical work week.

It is well known that people who are sleep deprived have impaired memory functioning. (2) We now know that your brain processes information without your awareness as well as when you are sleeping. This ability of the brain to process information is thought to contribute to your memory when you are awake. Specifically, memory for facts and knowledge is consolidating or coming together when we are sleeping.

However, as is often the case, the research is not completely clear. For example, we are not sure whether sleep deprivation affects working memory or our temporary storage and manipulation of information. This ability is important for such complex brain tasks as understanding language, learning, and reasoning.

In a recent study of more than 250 people published in the *Journal of Experimental Psychology*: General, Michigan State University researchers found that people derive vastly different effects from this "sleep memory" ability, with some memories improving dramatically and others not at all.

In an earlier study by other researchers published in *Current Directions in Psychological Science*, scientists found that sleep helps consolidate memories by fixing them in the brain. Thus, we are much better able to retrieve memories later on if we have gotten a good night's sleep.

This research suggests that sleep also helps us to reorganize memories, picking out the emotional details and reconfiguring the memories. The study revealed that sleep helps us to produce new and creative ideas and thinking. This means that problem solving improves with sleep quality.

In another study that appeared in the June 2012 issue in Nature Neuroscience, researchers found that subjects who were practicing a piece of music and heard it again while they were sleeping actually played it more accurately the next time. In that study there were 16 subjects with a range of music education who had learned to play two different melodies by pressing keys in time to the sequence of circular motion such as seen in the video game *Guitar Hero*.

The subjects in the study then took a 90-minute nap which allowed them to go through one normal sleep cycle which we will discuss later. One of the musical tunes was played over and over during the slow-wave sleep cycle period. Later, when the participants in the study were awake, they were better able to play both of the musical tunes. What is interesting about this particular study is that slow-wave sleep was shown to be important to memory consolidation. Thus, if you are not getting into those deeper levels of sleep, you are likely to have difficulties consolidating memory.

Consolidation refers to the fixing of memories that can occur whether we are awake or, as found in the recent research just noted, when we are sleeping. We now know that we can improve upon what we have learned during sleep. This is referred to as enhancement. You can improve your learning by making sure that you maintain a good sleep schedule.

Neuroscientists have discovered that it takes approximately six hours to consolidate something new. Thus, if you have learned something and it's important for you to remember it, don't take up a new activity within the same context. Rather, we now know that sleeping on what you've learned actually will improve and refresh brain circuits.

Sleep experts are not generally proponents of naps. (3) The reason for this is that the time that you spend sleeping during the day time (in the form of a nap) will take away from your sleep at night time. Thus, if you are having difficulty sleeping at night or sleeping through the night, you should avoid naps, if possible. However, if your sleep is generally in good shape, you may benefit from a nap.

Some people call these "power naps." I have a psychologist friend Dr. Robert Fisher who takes a 20-minute "power nap" usually at least once a day. He swears by these naps, and he tells me that they help him feel refreshed and that, as a consequence, he is much more productive.

The research would suggest that my friend is correct. (4) In fact, some research indicates that a power nap is nearly as effective as a memory enhancer as is a night's sleep. Learning words, facts, concepts, and being more creative are also improved.

Regardless of the value of short naps, which I think is substantial, it's important to remember that if you sleep more than approximately 30 minutes, you are likely to interfere with your sleep cycle at night because you will be getting into the deeper levels of sleep and REM sleep during the daytime. Thus, make sure your "power naps" are less than 30 minutes.

So in summary, naps can enhance your consolidation of memory, increase your creative juices, and power up and enhance the brain circuits involved in learning and memory retention. (2)

These recent studies reinforced the results of the first study to show that sleep protects memories from interference. That first study was reported by Jeffrey Ellenbogen, MD, Harvard Medical School, at the 2007 59th Annual Meeting of the American Academy of Neurology. **Simply put, sleep deprived people don't remember as much.**

The research studies have provided important insights into how the sleeping brain interacts with memories: it appears to strengthen them. Thus, one of the things that we have found challenging in our assessment and diagnosis of people with mild traumatic brain injury is ferreting out what is the result of the brain injury itself and what might be the result of sleep deprivation in the case where sleep problems exist.

Perhaps then, sleep disorders might worsen memory problems seen in people with dementia but also those individuals who are experiencing memory problems for other reasons including concussion.

All in all, it would appear that sleep hygiene, or methods and procedures to help people sleep better, will also have protective effects on memory. Perhaps the quote by the Dalai Lama says it best: "Sleep is the best meditation."

What is Insomnia?

Insomnia is a common type of sleep disorder that millions of Americans experience. If you have insomnia, you have trouble falling asleep, staying asleep, or both. You may also wake up too early in the morning. You may get too little sleep, or your quality of sleep may be poor. It's not uncommon for people with insomnia to be able to sleep through the night but awaken in the morning feeling fatigued. This would be an example of poor sleep quality, and, of course, it could have many causes.

Insomnia can be short lived or acute. For example, you may have experienced a divorce or death in the family and been unable to sleep. You may have been traveling and sleeping in an unfamiliar environment and are not sleeping well. These would be examples of acute sleep problems that will resolve when the stressor dissipates or the life circumstance changes.

When we think of "acute insomnia," we are describing a condition that lasts for several days or several weeks. Conversely, chronic insomnia lasts for one month or more. In fact, there are people who have been experiencing insomnia for years; we would call this a severe and stubborn type of chronic insomnia. Whether you decide to seek professional help or try to work through your insomnia on your own, you will probably relate in part to the length of time you have been experiencing the sleep disturbance.

There are three common forms of insomnia: Sleep onset insomnia means the person is having difficulty falling asleep at their designated bedtime. Sleep maintenance means that the person wakes up during the night and has trouble falling back asleep. If you wake up in the night and have trouble falling back asleep within 10 or 15 minutes, you are likely experiencing some type of sleep maintenance problem.

Terminal insomnia refers to awakening too early in the morning. If you have set your alarm for 7 a.m. but awaken at 6 o'clock, and if this occurs frequently, you're having terminal insomnia. The types of interventions that you employ in part relate to the type of insomnia that you are experiencing.

When a doctor renders the diagnosis of insomnia it basically comes down to the question of **primary** or **secondary** insomnia.

Most cases involving chronic insomnia can be traced to a symptom or side effect of some other type of difficulty that the person is experiencing. Thus, we call it secondary insomnia. Secondary insomnia would be due to some type of medical condition, difficulties associated with medication, and other substances that may cause secondary insomnia. If the insomnia is secondary, the question becomes should it be treated?

Primary insomnia is not due to some type of medical condition, medication, or other types of substances that the person is exposed to. Rather, primary insomnia is its own separate distinct disorder, and unfortunately the causes of primary insomnia are not well understood. What we do know is that long-lasting stressors, significant environmental problems, and emotional upset can cause primary insomnia.

It's also possible for a secondary insomnia to develop into a primary insomnia. For example, if the original medical condition has resolved itself and the person continues to experience insomnia, they may have developed a primary insomnia which now needs treatment.

Is My Sleep Normal?

In order for us to understand sleep problems, we really should start by understanding what represents "normal" sleep. This has been studied for many years. Sleep researchers believe that most adults require at least seven hours of sleep per night. As with most things in life, there is variability. Some people need very little sleep in order to function adequately, but they are certainly in the minority. Another group of people may need 10 to 12 hours of sleep to function normally. They would also be considered to be in the minority. Generally seven or eight hours of sleep is sufficient for most people.

The need for sleep can also vary related to age. Children and adolescents need more sleep and also require naps until at least the age of five. The National Sleep Foundation provides the following guidelines for sleep:

- Newborns (1–2 months): 10.5 to 18 hours per day
- Infants (3–11 months): 9–12 hours (daytime naps of 30 to 120 minutes are common)

- Toddlers (1–3 years): 12–14 hours per day (naps gradually decrease to 1 to 3 hours)
- Preschoolers (3–5 years): 11–13 hours (naps after age 5 are less common)
- School-aged (5–12 years): 10–11 hours

Sleep and Rhythms

We will try and limit the technical terms in this section, but it is helpful to understand how your body clock and sleep relate.

Circadian rhythms are regular changes in thinking and physical characteristics that occur in the course of a 24-hour period or day. (Circadian is Latin for "around a day.") Most circadian rhythms are regulated by the body's biological "clock."

This clock, or the SCN (suprachiasmatic nucleus), is actually a pair of pinhead-sized brain structures that together contain about 20,000 brain cells or neurons. The SCN rests in the hypothalamus, a part of the brain known for memory processing. This part of the brain is just above the point where the vision nerve tracts cross or in the middle part of the brain. (Recently it was discovered that there are photoreceptors in the retina at the back of the eye. Light travels from these nerve cells along the optic nerve to the SCN.)

Signals from the SCN travel to various areas of the brain, including the pineal gland. This part of the brain responds to light-induced signals by turning off production of the hormone melatonin.

You will see from our following discussion on nutrition that melatonin is very involved in sleep and can also be stimulated by certain foods. The body's level of melatonin normally increases as night approaches, making people feel drowsy. We call this sleep inertia.

The SCN also regulates functions that are coordinated with the sleep/wake cycle. These activities include your body temperature, secretion of certain hormones, changes in your blood pressure, and the making of urine.

Research scientists have learned that most people's biological clocks work on a 25-hour cycle rather than a 24-hour one. (5) However, because sunlight and bright lights can reset the SCN, our biological cycles normally follow the 24-hour cycle of the sun, rather than our internal cycle with which we were born.

Circadian rhythms can be disrupted somewhat by modern-day stimuli, which might include your alarm clock, the sound of an engine, or the schedule of your meals. For example, when traveling you should always eat your first meal in the new time zone and not before. This will help you recover from moving through the various time zones that results in jet lag.

Jet lag can also be manipulated by light therapy. Exposure to special lights that are many times brighter than the ordinary light in your home helps to reset the biological clock and adjust to a new time zone.

These special lights can also help you be alert at other times. For example, if you have trouble getting started in the morning because you have to get up particularly early, eating your breakfast while sitting under one of these lights would likely help you become alert more quickly.

Symptoms similar to jet lag are common in people who work nights or who perform shift work. Because the schedules are opposed to the powerful sleep-regulating cues like sunlight, they often become uncontrollably drowsy during work.

Are you a shift worker? Shift workers may suffer insomnia or other problems when they try to sleep. Studies have shown that shift workers have an increased risk of behavioral health problems, heart disease, and digestive disturbances which correlate to their sleeping problems. Thus, if you are a shift worker, it's extremely important that you follow the guidelines in this book. You also may be one of those people who regularly benefit from a power nap as described earlier.

Also of great concern from a public health perspective are the number and seriousness of accidents in the workplace. Incidents or accidents have been shown to increase during the night shift. Night-shift workers have been found to be, at least in part, responsible for major accidents such as the Exxon Valdez oil spill, Three Mile Island, and the Chernobyl nuclear power plant accident.

Still other research has found that medical interns working on the night shift **are two times more likely** as others to misinterpret hospital test records. Obviously, this could lead to errors which endanger patient care. Some have suggested that installing bright lights, minimizing the number of shift changes, and scheduling naps may decrease work-related accidents. These are general guidelines that you may also wish to consider as you improve your sleep and overall brain health.

Do I Have a Sleep Problem?

Before we begin, it will be beneficial for you to take a self-test to determine the extent of your sleep problems. This assessment is not designed to replace an assessment by your

healthcare provider, but it can be a starting point to help you begin to solve your sleep problems on your own. Also, if you decide to seek professional help, you will be able to provide your healthcare provider with more specific information about your insomnia.

Accurate and specific data about any health problem is essential for healthcare providers to provide you with effective solutions to you problems. Go to the following website, complete the questionnaire, and then come back to continue our work.

http://www.londonsleepcentre.com/sleepdisorders/onlinequestion naire.htm

What is Memory?

In psychology, memory involves the brain functions used to store, retain, and recall information and experiences. However, scientists have refined this definition in different ways.

Memory has various parts. You can have memory of what you see, hear, touch, and smell. There is short-term, intermediate, and long-term memory. There is also working memory, meaning the act of holding things in your brain temporarily while you manipulate it.

It is possible for you to be very good at one type of memory process and yet do poorly at another. In fact, during my assessment of people who have a suspected brain injury, I will frequently find that one type of memory might be much more effective than another type of memory. People tend to think of memory as global. In fact, there are many different types of memory. Because the scope of this book is focused on methods to help you sleep better and to improve your memory and health, we will not engage in a comprehensive discussion of memory here.

If you have an interest in learning much more about memory and especially improving your memory and brain health, you will want to obtain our other book Brain Health: Simple Steps to a Better Memory. In that book, as well as on my website, we discuss the various types of memory—of which there are many.

Follow these links for information:

http://www.amazon.com/BrainHealthSimpleBetterebook/dp/B00
8S9A9I8

http://www.memory-loss-facts.com

How Does Sleep Affect Memory?

Sleep-deprived people don't perform well, and people are sleeping less every year. According to the National Sleep Foundation, 63 percent of Americans report that they do not meet their need for sleep during a typical work week.

It is well known that people who are sleep deprived have impaired memory functioning. There is substantial research evidence proving that your brain is processing information without your awareness. This ability of the brain to process information is thought to contribute to your memory in a waking state. Specifically, sleep-dependent declarative memory—or more simply put, memory for facts and knowledge—is in consolidation when we are sleeping.

However, as is often the case, the research is not completely clear. For example, we are not sure whether sleep deprivation affects working memory. Working memory refers to our temporary storage and manipulation of the information. This ability is important for such complex brain or thinking tasks as language comprehension, learning, and reasoning.

In a recent study of more than 250 people published in the *Journal of Experimental Psychology: General,* Michigan State University researchers found that people derive vastly different effects from this "sleep memory" ability, with some memories improving dramatically and others not at all. (6)

In an earlier study by other researchers published in Current Directions in Psychological Science, scientists found that sleep helps consolidate memories by fixing them in the brain. (7) Thus, we can retrieve memories later much better if we have gotten a good night's sleep.

This research suggested that sleep also helps us to reorganize memories, picking out the emotional details and reconfiguring the memories. The study revealed that this sleep helps us to produce new and creative ideas and thinking. This means that problem solving improves with sleep quality.

These recent studies also reinforced the results of Ellenbogen's study (reported in 2007) to show that sleep protects memories from interference. Simply put, sleep deprived people don't remember as much.

The research studies have provided important insights into how the sleeping brain interacts with memories: it appears to strengthen them. Perhaps, then, sleep disorders might worsen memory problems seen in people with dementia.

Consequently, it would appear that sleep hygiene (methods and procedures to help people sleep better) will also have protective effects on memory. Perhaps the quote by the Dalai Lama says it best: "Sleep is the best meditation."

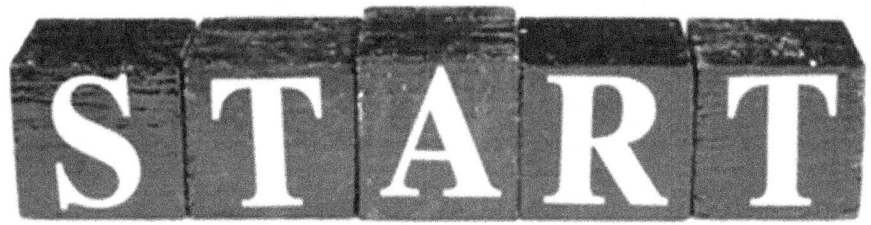

Quick Start Guide – Sleep Better Tonight

We know from research that sleep deprivation can affect memory consolidation in the brain. As a neuropsychologist who attempts to identify the causes of memory loss in my practice daily, loss of sleep is always a consideration. Here are the things research has shown that you can do now to improve your chance of sleeping better tonight and every night going forward. (3, 8) Follow these principles for better sleep and brain health.

Principle 1: Pick a Regular Wake-up Time

Changes in your sleep-wake schedule can upset your sleep. In fact, you can create the type of sleep problem that occurs in jet lag by changing your wake-up time from day-to-day or week-to-week. If you stick to a regular wake-up time, you will soon notice that you are becoming sleepy at about the right time each night to allow you to get the sleep you need.

Principle 2: The Bed Is Only for Sleeping

While in bed, you should refrain from doing things that you do when you are awake. Do not read, watch TV, eat, problem solve, study, argue, use the phone, or do other things that require you to be awake while you are in bed.

If you often use your bed for activities other than sleep, you are unintentionally teaching yourself to stay awake in bed. If you avoid these activities while in bed, your bed will ultimately become a place where it is easy to go to sleep. And you will stay asleep. Sexual activity is the only exception to principle number two.

Principle 3: When You Can't Sleep—Get Up

Never, ever stay in bed, either at the beginning of the night or during the middle of the night, for extended periods without being asleep.

More than 15 or 20 minutes of being awake in bed will usually lead to tossing and turning, becoming frustrated, or worrying about not sleeping. These reactions, in turn, make it more difficult to fall asleep and lead to sleep deprivation.

Also, if you lie in bed awake for long periods, you are teaching your brain to be awake in bed. When sleep does not come on or return quickly, it is best to get up, go to another room, and return to bed only when you feel sleepy enough to fall asleep quickly. You should get up if you find yourself awake for 15 or 20 minutes or so and you do not feel as though you are about to go to sleep.

Principle 4: Avoid Worry or Problem Solving in Bed

Do not anguish, mull over your problems, plan future actions, or do other problem solving or thinking while in bed. These actions, we have determined, are negative or bad mental habits. If your mind seems to be racing or you can't seem to shut off your thinking, get out of bed and go to another room.

When you feel that you can return to bed without your thinking interrupting your sleep, give it a try. If this disruptive thinking occurs often, you should routinely set aside a time early each evening to do the thinking, worrying, problem solving, and/or planning you need to do. If you start this method, you will have fewer intrusive thoughts while you are in bed.

Principle 5: No Daytime Napping

You should avoid all daytime napping. If you must nap, do so for no more than 30 minutes so that you don't get involved in the 90-minute sleep cycle. Sleeping during the day partially satisfies your sleep needs and, thus, will reduce your drive to sleep at night.

Principle 6: When You Are Sleepy, Go to Bed, but Not before the Time You Have Set

Generally speaking, you should go to bed when you feel sleepy to avoid developing more sleep debt. However, do not go to bed so early that you are spending far more time in bed each night that you need for sleep. Too much time in bed results in a fragmented or broken sleep. If you spend too much time in bed, you probably will make your sleep problem worse.

If these first-line, non-medicine approaches do not work, you may need a sleep study. Medication can help but is not recommended as a long-term approach.

GOOD HEALTH - GOOD HEALTH

Exercise +
Sleep +
Outdoor life +
Prevention +
Relax
Medical Checks +
Good hygiene +
No drugs +
Sport activity +
No smoking +
Healthy diet =

—————————————————

GOOD HEALTH

Does Sleep Deprivation Affect My Physical Health?

Obesity and Sleep Loss

Authorities have some new weight-loss advice that's sure to be welcome news: Sleep can be just as influential to a successful diet as healthful eating and exercise.

"Chronic sleep restriction is pervasive in modern societies, and there is robust evidence supporting the role of reduced sleep as contributing to the current obesity epidemic," writes a team of obesity experts in a recent edition of the *Canadian Medical Association Journal.* (9)

The evidence includes findings that fatigued brains prompt people to consume more, and that some hormones that regulate appetite and metabolism don't work correctly in people who don't get enough sleep.

The authors of the *CMAJ* analysis cite an experiment reported in the Annals of Internal Medicine in 2010. Two groups of obese adults were put on a diet then forced to cut 680 calories per day from their diets. Additionally, one group slept for eight and a half hours per night and the other slept only a half hour per night. After two weeks, study participants in the sleep-deprived group had lost 55 percent less body fat than their well-rested counterparts.

Further, they lost 60 percent more lean body mass. The authors of the study concluded that when the body is sleep deprived, holding on to fat becomes a priority.

The authors of the study conducted their own investigation with 12 dieting adults. After 17 weeks, sleep habits were able to predict the quantity of fat loss, they wrote.

In another study, the researchers traced the link between weight and sleep in adults over the course of six years. At the end of the experiment, people who got seven to eight hours of sleep per night gained five pounds less than people who slept fewer than six hours per night.

The bottom line is that sleep is a critical item in your list of variables that needs to be reviewed when you are focused upon a weight-management program.

High Blood Pressure

New research indicates that those with high blood pressure who struggle to get enough sound sleep are twice as likely to have an unyielding case of hypertension as those who sleep well.

Studying more than 230 patients with high blood pressure, scientists from the University of Pisa in Italy also found that women scored much higher than men on measures of insomnia, and most participants slept six or fewer hours per night. The subjects in the study had an average age of 58. (10)

"There are a number of studies demonstrating a relationship between hypertension risk and insomnia and short sleep duration, but no one correlated poor sleep quality with hypertension severity [before]," said study author Rosa Maria Bruno, a doctoral student and research fellow at the Institute of Clinical Physiology-National Council of Research in Pisa.

The results of Bruno's study suggest that insomnia in complicated hypertensive patients, particularly females, could be clinically relevant not only for quality of life but also for cardiovascular health and should not be disregarded.

About 75 million people in the United States have diagnosed high blood pressure. Approximately 50 million people take anti-hypertensive medications. But drugs alone don't sufficiently control the condition—a major risk factor for cardiovascular disease—in 20 to 30 percent of those cases, according to the American Heart Association.

High blood pressure is considered unyielding if patients are taking three or more hypertension drugs but still have blood pressure readings higher than 140/90 mmHg.

Although short-sleep duration was highly prevalent in all subjects in the study, women were found to suffer out of proportion from poor sleep quality and depressive symptoms. About 12 percent of the subjects in the study had experienced previous cardiovascular events, while 8 percent had diabetes and 15 percent were also smokers.

The researchers concluded that there is evidence that sleep and cardiovascular disorders are tightly linked. But, as with all research, more study is necessary with various populations. Regardless, sleep problems also are related to obesity and diabetes, which contribute to resistance to blood-pressure-lowering drugs.

Researchers have concluded that living with a chronic disease, like resistant hypertension, likely act as a chronic stressor, causing disruption of sleep.

The research clearly indicates that good sleep habits, including getting regular exercise as we have discussed elsewhere in this book, will most likely promote peaceful sleep.

Many of us are all wired up in day-to-day life. Stress is a part of life and we are all exposed to multiple stressors in our lives. Our bodies react to those stressors by releasing hormones and other chemicals that make the organs work harder.

If we have insomnia, we're not getting rest for those organs and eventually they'll start malfunctioning. The bottom line is that the only way to help our bodies is by getting enough hours of sleep and also good quality sleep.

Parkinson's Disease and Sleep

Parkinson's disease (PD) is a neurological disorder caused by a deficit of the neurotransmitter dopamine in the brain and primarily affects movement. (11) This disease is most common in men and symptoms tend to begin after age 50. However, there are cases where it is diagnosed in younger adults.

The unintentional movements that the PD patient makes can contribute to poor sleep quality. People with PD sometimes have poor memory. But what is also problematic, as we have discussed elsewhere in this book, is that sleep deprivation or poor sleep quality can also affect the memory of those with PD.

PD is a chronic progressive disease, though the course of Parkinson's disease varies in severity and the timeline of the progression of symptoms.

There are some promising areas of research in finding the causes of Parkinson's disease and possible cures. Scientists have identified some genetic markers and links to this disease. Experiments involving stem-cell transplantation have shown promise in alleviating the motor symptoms of the disorder, but this research is still ongoing and has not been tested successfully in humans as of yet.

The onset of Parkinson's disease is gradual and subtle. There is no diagnostic test for the disease. A doctor will make a diagnosis based upon the results of a comprehensive medical history and neurological examination. The physician might also order brain images or various laboratory tests to rule out other diseases.

Basically the symptoms are classified in the following clusters:

- Tremors of hands, arms, legs, and feet
- Balance and coordination impairment
- Slowness of movement
- Stiffness of arms and legs

Other symptoms that might occur with Parkinson's disease include depression, anxiety, and other emotional issues; problems with chewing, swallowing, talking, and incontinence may also occur.

What treatments are available for Parkinson's disease?

Treatment and symptom management is the key to helping the PD patient sleep better at night. Avoiding sleep deprivation or building a sleep debt will also improve memory and overall brain health.

There are a number of medications used to treat the symptoms of this disorder. Levadopa, the chemical predecessor of dopamine, is often prescribed along with carbidopa to treat slowness in movements and muscle rigidity.

Anticholinergic medications are used to treat muscle tremors. Other medications that are prescribed because they mimic the neurotransmitter dopamine include   bromocriptine, pramipexole, and ropinole.

In the event medication is not effective in managing involuntary movements and tremors that affect sleep and other symptoms, a surgical intervention called **Deep Brain Stimulation (DBS)** might be recommended by the treating physician.

DBS involves placing electrodes deep into the brain; these electrodes are connected to a device that generates small electrical impulses, in some ways similar to a TENS unit. Studies show this intervention provides some symptomatic relief, but this intervention does not cure Parkinson's disease. However, if the PD patient has some relief, we may see an improvement in sleep quality.

In summary, Parkinson's disease can affect sleep because of the involuntary movements associated with the disease. Medication to manage the symptoms of PD offers hope to those with the disease in managing the symptoms previously mentioned. Following the guidelines in the book for proper sleep hygiene can play an important role in symptom management as well. With improved sleep the potential effects of PD on memory loss may be mitigated.

Diabetes and Sleep

Research reported in Science Daily in 2008 suggested that reducing slow-wave or deep sleep in otherwise healthy people has the effect of disturbing the regulation of glucose (sugar) levels. (12) Thus, the researchers concluded that the risk of Type II diabetes increases with poor sleep quality and especially slow-wave sleep deprivation.

What is slow-wave sleep? As discussed earlier, this relates to the Stage IV sleep level in our sleep cycle. A variety of studies have indicated that reduced sleep quality affects the metabolism or use of glucose and regulation of appetite in people. The result is an increased risk of obesity and diabetes from sleep deprivation. Some patients in research studies actually gained 20 to 30 pounds because of this poor regulation of sleep. Research on this topic is ongoing at various universities, including the University of Chicago and other sites funded by the National Institutes of Health. It is prudent to get better deep sleep to avoid the potentially devastating effects on glucose metabolism this type of sleep deprivation can cause.

Understanding diabetes can be hard, even for people who have suffered from it their whole lives. Finding the right resources to become educated on the topic can be even harder. You, on the other hand, are in luck. You are about to read a segment dedicated to help you comprehend what diabetes is all about. In this way, you will also be able to manage your sleep and ultimately your brain health more effectively.

Diabetes does not have many symptoms, and when you do not take your medications, there is often no immediate effect. However, it is very dangerous as untreated diabetes can easily lead to more dangerous health conditions, such as heart disease. If you have diabetes, make sure to stay vigilant about taking your medications to prevent further complications, including the development of sleep and memory problems.

When following a diabetic diet, understand that you can make certain exchanges to prevent becoming bored with your diet and being tempted to "cheat." Foods on a diabetic diet are categorized as proteins, fats, and carbohydrates. You will be given lists of these foods, and you can exchange one for another of equal values. For example, you could have half a cup of cooked pasta, or a small baked or boiled potato, or a slice of bread but not all of these at once.

Although it may seem rather depressing when you find out that you have been diagnosed with diabetes, know that you can still continue living the life you have been leading with a few minor tweaks. You should meet with a nutritionist that will help adjust the diet you are used to.

Go online for help with your diabetes! I am a big advocate of support groups and communities. There are many forums and groups of people who are just like you, and they love to help others. You'll find all kinds of advice about every facet of diabetic life, from coping with family members who are not supportive to recipes and diet tips.

When you combine smoking and diabetes, blood vessel damage to your extremities can increase significantly. Blood pressure often increases, resulting in damage to small blood vessels in the feet and hands and impairing blood flow. This can result in reduced circulation, which, in turn, can result in ulcers, particularly on the feet. Blood vessels in the brain can also be impacted, contributing to attention and memory problems.

As was stated in the beginning of this section, diabetes is a hard condition for people to comprehend, including those who have it. With this information we've just provided, you are on your way to becoming educated about diabetes. Use this advice to help you learn how to cope with diabetes, improve your brain health, and enhance your sleep.

Effects of Poor Sleep on Psychological Health

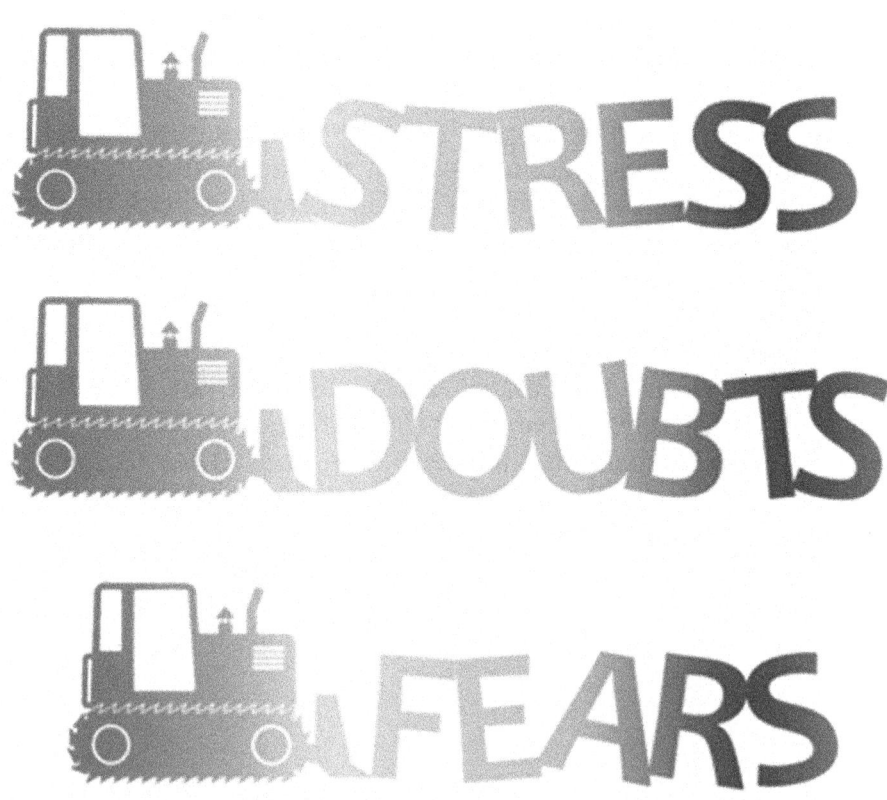

In this section we will discuss the relationship between sleep and anxiety and anxiety and sleep. Anxiety has long been recognized as a factor in preventing sleep. But ongoing insomnia can also lead to the development of anxiety, particularly an anxiety where the person anticipates and fears insomnia. Let's get started.

Anxiety and Worry

Anxiety affects sleep and sleep affects anxiety. (13) When you are anxious during the day, you are more likely to carry those anxieties into your bedroom at night. If you are having difficulty sleeping at night, you may develop anticipatory anxiety. In other words, you become anxious as bedtime approaches as you believe you may not be able to sleep once again. Anxiety is a major contributor to sleep loss.

Anxiety is an issue that many people have to deal with today. Oftentimes, unnecessary worry leads to a lot of stress and causes you to feel anxious. You need to change the way you think in order to help avoid stressful issues. The following section contains a number of helpful tips to get you to think more positively. Thinking more positively will help you avoid anxiety as a barrier to sleeping better tonight and into the future.

When should I seek professional help for anxiety?

If your anxiety causes you to self-medicate, decreases the quality or length of your sleep, or causes you to consider harming yourself, medical attention is necessary. A therapist, counselor, or psychiatrist can help you to create a treatment plan to alleviate your anxiety and keep you from hurting yourself. If you believe that professional help is necessary, contact your state psychological association for a referral to a qualified professional.

As a clinical and neuropsychologist, I have a bias toward my profession. However, many social workers have been trained as therapists as well. The main thing is that you connect with a therapist skilled in working with anxiety.

Use humor to combat your anxiety. Laughter can be extremely helpful for clearing your mind when you're having an anxiety attack. Try reading jokes from some funny books or watching some funny television or movies. Soon, you'll be on your way to feeling more relieved and relaxed so that you can stop the attack.

Reduce your level of anxiety by asking others for help when you need it. Many people feel that asking for help is a sign of weakness, but it is actually a very intelligent thing to do when a task is more than you can handle. Delegating appropriate tasks to others will keep anxiety under control.

Spend as much time as possible enjoying friends and family. Laughter has been called "the best medicine," and there is lots of truth to that. Plan an evening or an outing with those you love at least once a week, and you will have something to look forward to the rest of the time.

Learn how to distract yourself. As soon as you feel the anxiety starting to overwhelm you, find something that offers a distraction. Make sure that it's something that takes up a lot of concentration or energy, such as a difficult puzzle or a brisk workout. By concentrating on something other than your anxiety, you will find that it disappears quite quickly.

Laughter is one of the very best ways to circumvent anxiety because it changes your focus and lightens your mood. As a tension breaker it cannot be beat, and the best part is that its effects can be shared with those around you. Try to cultivate an appreciation for the silly and absurd side of life. Embrace the funny and witty people in your life. Bring them closer so that their resilience becomes a model for you.

Sometimes, there is no easy way to deal with anxiety and simple home remedies may not work for you. In these cases, it is highly advisable that you seek help from a professional therapist or physician and ask about what types of medication may be beneficial to your needs. This should be looked at as a last resort. And be careful that you don't become dependent on benzodiazepines like Xanax, Ativan, or Valium.

Anxiety can be caused by many different factors, so it is important to understand the root causes before trying to treat them. If you are unable to pinpoint exactly why you are feeling anxious, you will be unable to learn how to remove this anxiety with an easy and quick method.

Keep yourself as busy as possible at all times. When you have down time, it will be easier for your mind to focus on negative things and will, therefore, fuel anxiety. Start your day out by cleaning the house, working in the garden, reading a book, or doing some other activity that you enjoy.

When you are on anxiety medication, **never stop taking it without talking to your doctor.** Even if you feel like you are better, you still cannot just stop. Some of these medications can make you very ill and can even be deadly if you just stop taking them all of a sudden.

A great way to address anxiety is to **master the art of diaphragmatic breathing.** When you have the ability to focus on this type of deep breathing from the stomach, it is possible to achieve a sense of calm and contentedness that can calm even the most stressful of situations.

To learn a valuable deep-breathing technique that can help you combat anticipatory anxiety about sleep, visit this YouTube site:

http://www.youtube.com/watch?v=-j5Z4E2wkh4&feature=related

Find some reasons to laugh at the world. You can watch a funny movie or television show, and this will also take your mind off of any worries you might have. So find a comedy on the television, sit back, and do not forget to let out those laughs.

A lot of people today experience anxiety. Anxiety is the enemy of a good night's rest. To help rid yourself of anxiety and sleep better, you should use the power of positive thinking.

By believing that the events in your life will only turn out negative, this mindset will cause you undue amounts of worry. Therefore, if you are going to be less stressed and more calm, you need to change your thought processes and soon. If you focus on combating what I call "stinken thinken" you will see your anxiety begin to fade away and disappear.

The Worry System

Research has indicated that identifying problems and generating possible solutions can help you sleep better at night. (3) Clinicians have found it very effective for people to schedule their problem solving and worry several hours before bedtime. Simply select a time at least three hours before bedtime. Sit down in a quiet environment. Use the following Worry Form.

Worry Form

Concern #1   Solution #1

                                              Solution #2

	Solution #3
Concern #2	Solution #1
	Solution #2
	Solution #3

Etcetera

Step One: Identify one or more concerns that have been intruding into your mind at night.

Step Two: Without filtering, generate as many possible solutions as you can. Don't edit as you go along as this will stifle your creativity. Just simply write them down on the form above as they come into your mind.

Step Three: Now choose one of the solutions that may be helpful to solving the concern. Decide when and how you will implement the solution.

Step Four: Repeat the first three steps. Usually people will have two to four worries that have been affecting their sleep.

Step Five: When you go to bed, use the breathing technique previously noted. Imagine in your mind's eye a relaxing scene (perhaps a place you have been in the past or a place you would like to be that you think of as calming and safe) as you practice the breathing.

Step Six: If one of the concerns intrudes into your mind, remind yourself of the solution that you selected earlier in the evening. Go back to relaxed breathing and your relaxing image on the movie screen.

IMPORTANT:

Do not push thoughts or images out of your mind. Instead, simply let them travel across the movie screen in your mind. Return to the breathing technique. Remind yourself as needed of your solution that you generated earlier in the evening for the concern.

Many of my patients have had great success using this technique to avoid taking their worries and concerns into the bedroom. It takes a little practice, but it works if you are consistent. It only takes 15 minute earlier in the evening and works in most cases. Give it a try; you will be happy you did.

Depression and Insomnia

Depression is very serious problem that can contribute to sleep problems in a significant way. (14, 15) Depression can make functioning seem impossible. It can impair every aspect of your life and make simple things like getting out of bed and eating seem very hard to do.

According to the World Health Organization (WHO), depression is one of the major illnesses when ranked by its impact on productivity. Depression directly affects 121 million people worldwide.

According to the Centers for Disease Control and Prevention, we now know that sleep apnea is a risk factor for depression. The CDC reviewed the medical records of 10,000 people in the United States who have been diagnosed with sleep apnea. Men who were diagnosed with sleep apnea had twice the likelihood of developing depression. Even more startling was the fact that depression was five times more likely in women who suffer from sleep apnea. These findings were published in the April 2012 issue of Sleep.

We used to think of a sleep disorder as secondary to or caused by something like depression. However, there is growing evidence that sleep deprivation itself, regardless of the cause, can result in symptoms of clinical depression. (15) Thus, not only is insomnia a symptom of depression but it can actually be a cause of depression. As we will see as we discuss other issues related to psychological and behavioral health, it has become increasingly clear that insomnia and sleep deprivation in and of itself is a separate disorder that needs attention from the healthcare community.

Just like anxiety, however, you can begin to feel depressed because you are sleep deprived. In other words, depression can result from poor sleep quality and sleep deprivation.

It is worth repeating that the relationship between sleep and depressive illness is complex—depression may cause sleep problems and sleep problems may cause or be partly responsible for depressive disorders.

For some people, symptoms of depression occur before the beginning of sleep problems. For others, sleep problems arrive first.

Sleep problems and depression may also share risk factors and biological features, and the two problems may respond to some of the same treatment strategies. Sleep problems are also affiliated with more severe depressive disorder.

If depression or frequent sadness is affecting your sleep, this segment will give you simple tips to deal with depression that you can use to help yourself sleep better at night.

Insomnia is very common among depressed people. According to the National Sleep Foundation, evidence suggests that people with insomnia have a ten-fold risk of developing depression when compared with individuals who sleep well.

Depressed individuals may suffer from a range of insomnia symptoms, including difficulty falling asleep (sleep onset insomnia), difficulty staying asleep (sleep maintenance insomnia), non-restorative sleep, and fatigability during the day. However, research has suggested that the risk of developing depression is topmost among people who suffer from both sleep onset and sleep maintenance insomnia.

According to the National Institutes of Health, depression may be described as feeling sad, blue, unhappy, miserable, or down in the dumps. Most of us feel this way at one time or another for short periods.

Clinical depression is a mood disorder in which feelings of sadness, loss, anger, or frustration interfere with everyday life for a longer period of time. Major depressive disorder is a condition that requires the intervention of a professional.

Signs and symptoms of depression include:

- Low or irritable mood most of the time
- A loss of enjoyment in usual daily activities
- As already noted, trouble sleeping or sleeping too much
- A big difference in appetite, associated with weight gain or loss
- Fatigue and lack of energy
- Feelings of low self-esteem, self-hate, and irrational guilt
- Difficulty attending and concentrating
- Sluggish or fast movements
- Little activity and avoiding usual activities
- Feeling hopeless or helpless

- Preoccupied with thoughts of death or suicide

If five or more of these listed symptoms have been present for at least two weeks, please consider seeking professional help. Contact a behavioral health professional who has experience with depression. Don't just rely on your family doctor to give you an antidepressant. Rather, ask for a referral to a specialist.

Medication can often help, but you should always try personal counseling as the first line of treatment. Once you go down the road of antidepressant medication, it may take awhile before you will be able to stop it. And it can take up to eight weeks for the medication to be effective.

Certainly mild depression, and especially depression associated with life events such as divorce or job loss, requires counseling first and not drugs (or psychopharmacology) as the first line of treatment.

As a practicing neuroscientist and behavioral health professional I have seen too many patients go down the road of medication prior to considering problem-solving approaches and personal counseling first. These patients are consequently on medication for many years and after time the brain adjusts to and requires the stimulation of serotonin by these medications.

Many experts believe that evidenced-based psychotherapy (e.g., Cognitive Behavioral Therapy (CBT) or Problem Solving Therapy (PST)) should be the first line of treatment for most forms of mild to moderate depression.

The following are some common methods to help improve mood and thus increase the likelihood of a good night's sleep. (16)

49

Develop a routine. Having an established routine can help lessen depression by keeping unwelcome surprises out of your life. Knowing what to expect in your life can help you feel better and more prepared to deal with any unexpected events. Having a good schedule and a back-up plan are great methods of preparation.

Eat a healthy diet. As we have discussed elsewhere in this book, good nutrition is fundamental to proper sleep. Many times someone who is depressed may try to cover those feelings with overeating, binge drinking, or even starving themselves.

Suppressed feelings are one of the largest contributing factors in depression. **When you find yourself reaching for the bag of cookies or bottle of wine, remind yourself that you are making the feelings worse.** In addition to forcing you to deal with your feelings instead of covering them, maintaining healthy eating habits will improve your health as well as your mood.

If you are feeling depressed, consider joining a church. Churches offer wonderful support networks and uplifting messages. They also offer a spiritual connection to a higher being, which can have a positive effect on a depressed state of mind. If you are unable to leave your home to reach a church, consider contacting one for a personal visit from the pastor to receive some of the same benefits.

A support group can provide a wonderful means of dealing with depression. Local support groups can be found on the Internet or are generally published one day a week in your daily newspaper.

Sometimes you might feel like you are the only one dealing with a particular problem. This is likely not true. A support group will connect you with individuals who have experienced what you are experiencing. It can provide a great outlet for your emotions and wonderful resources for coping too.

To combat feeling unmotivated, keep yourself moving by setting small goals with tangible rewards. This will enable you to enjoy the results of your hard work quicker and more frequently. Keeping small goals also means that the occasional missed goals will be easier to recover from, keeping your self-esteem high.

Know the symptoms of post-partum depression, and make sure that your partner does, too. While some "baby blues" are normal after giving birth, **post-partum depression is a serious, yet common illness that can benefit greatly from professional help.** Your partner can help you watch for signs that you need some help, as you may not be able to see the situation clearly yourself.

If you are facing depression at sub-clinical levels, you may want to try some over the counter remedies. For example, grape juice and St. John's wort have both been shown to have a positive impact on the mental welfare of their users. It is also cheaper than the more common prescription therapy. However, I don't advise St. John's wort unless you talk with your family doctor. (I once had a patient who was taking it and a prescription antidepressant, which also acted on serotonin in the brain. Thus, the person was overdosing without being aware.)

Go back to activities you used to enjoy, even if you don't feel like it. Push yourself at first, but it will get easier. Going through the motions of a fun activity, such as painting or playing a sport, can help you feel more energetic. You might find that you are truly enjoying the activity after all, once you get started.

Be aware that you are depressed. If you know that you are depressed and acknowledge it, you are less likely to beat yourself up over what you think you are doing wrong. Simply knowing that you are feeling depressed is sometimes enough to make you feel just a little bit better.

Even if you have never felt depressed before in your life, depression may emerge quickly and unexpectedly. Depression can have very late-stage onsets, so don't write it off even if you are in your forties or fifties. It can also strike both genders in almost equal amounts.

Becoming interested in the arts is a great way to help you beat your depression. If you like paintings or sculpture, be sure to schedule lots of visits to local museums. Likewise, if you like music, be sure to visit as many concerts and shows as you are able.

Create a social environment for yourself which will keep you from thinking negative thoughts. Call your friends together for an outing or gather family members for a social event. This helps you keep your negative and depressive attitude in check, while also surrounding yourself with positive people.

One way of dealing with depression is **to practice using positive visualization.** Start by closing your eyes and relaxing as much as possible. Take some deep breaths, and then begin imagining bright, happy scenes in your mind. For instance, if you love the outdoors, you could visualize yourself sitting by a beautiful stream with birds singing in the trees nearby. By choosing happy, uplifting scenes and then vividly imagining them, you can instantly lift your mood and begin feeling better.

Avoid caffeinated beverages such as coffee, tea, and soda. Besides the obvious effects on your sleep, caffeine has been shown to decrease the amount of serotonin in your brain, which can depress your mood. Caffeine will also make you jittery and anxious, adding to your depression. Importantly for our purpose in this book, caffeine can affect your sleep schedules, causing further problems with an already disrupted system.

If you have major depression, you should anticipate that many people won't be able to understand it. Most people think that depression is just like being really sad, but true sufferers know that this is not the truth. If people say things like "just chin up" to you, try to realize that they mean the best and just ignore it.

Take small steps. Depression can cause you to feel overwhelmed a lot of the time. By merely setting goals and doing a little bit at a time, you are sure to feel more in control. Another added benefit is that you can feel proud of yourself for taking those steps.

You have learned a lot of tips about dealing with depression. **Remember that this is not something that is going to go away overnight;** it will take some hard work and a lot of dedication. You can overcome depression. Even though it may seem impossible, it is not. Make sure you have the support that you need to get through this.

Anger, Irritability, and Poor Sleep

If you are harboring feelings of anger and irritability it is likely that your sleep may be affected. It is not uncommon for people to take their daytime feelings into their sleep. This not only applies to worry, anxiety, and depression but also to feelings of agitation or anger that have been unresolved.

The amygdala in the brain is the center for anger as well as anxiety. The front of the brain or the frontal lobes of the brain are responsible for mitigating and regulating feelings of anger and anxiety. If these two parts of the brain are not working together, there can be an increase in anger and anxiety symptoms that can contribute to sleep problems and deprivation. Likewise, sleep deprivation in and of itself can result in these two particular systems working less well.

If your irritability or feelings of anger are time limited, it is likely that they will resolve and not affect your sleep in a chronic or more lasting way. However, if you have been experiencing ongoing feelings of anger and a low tolerance for frustration for more than a week or two, you may need to seek professional guidance.

Our society requires that we communicate our feelings appropriately and without malice. If you are angry on a frequent basis, you are likely to alienate people in your personal life as well as those in the community. If your anger gets out of control, you may even get into legal trouble. Thus, managing anger goes well beyond the problems associated with it, causing insomnia and resulting in you having poor performance or brain functioning during the day because of sleep deprivation caused by persistent anger.

You may wish to consider the following questions suggested by the National Institutes of Health. When you experience an angry episode, ask yourself the following questions:

1. What was the first sign that I was angry?
2. What was it that triggered my anger?
3. How did I respond to this circumstance or situation?
4. What did I do well this time?
5. What can I do the next time this event occurs to handle it better?

If you ask yourself these questions each and every time you have an angry episode, you may find that your feelings of anger begin to diminish. You may also wish to consider some of the relaxation methods we discussed elsewhere in this book. Being able to manage your thoughts and your feelings around the issues that trigger anger will help you sleep better. If you are sleeping better, you will be more able to manage your stress, frustrations, and circumstances in your daily life that may contribute to stimulation of your amygdala. In short you will be using the front part of your brain or the frontal lobe to more effectively manage your feelings of anger.

Relationships and Sleep Problems

Most of us are aware that if our relationships are not functioning very well, we may not be sleeping well at night. However, it is much less common for us to be aware that our sleep deprivation or sleep problems are actually contributing to a relationship problem or conflict. Think back to the last time you had a conflict with your spouse, friend, or significant other. How did you sleep? Was your sleep affected by this conflict? How did your sleep differ if the conflict was ongoing?

Like most of the issues discussed in this section, sleep can affect relationships and poor relationships can affect sleep. Some of the reasons that have been identified as contributing to sleep disturbance in relationships are addressed in the following questions. Let's do a self-check.

1. Do you or your partner frequently move around in bed and thus cause the other to be in a lighter sleep?
2. Even worse, does your partner kick you in your sleep and wake you up?
3. You may notice that your partner snores and this awakens you in the middle of the night. Snoring is discussed elsewhere in the book.
4. Does each of you like the room temperature to be different? Does one of you like it to be hot and the other likes it to be cold?

5. Is there a lot of activity that goes on in your bedroom including TV watching, reading, keeping a light on low, and listening to music? Do any of these things affect your partner?
6. Do you and your partner have a different sleep schedule? She is a nurse and begins work at 7 a.m., but you don't have to be to the office until nine. Going to bed at different times or awakening at different times can cause some disruption in either of your sleep quality.
7. Does one of you generate a lot of heat, keeping the other away in bed? On the other hand, do you like to be close to your partner?
8. Do you frequently awaken during the night in order to go to the bathroom? Does this cause your partner to awaken or to be in a lighter sleep? Is it possible that they do not awaken but consequently they are fatigued in the morning because of poor sleep quality?

Did you answer yes to one or more of the above questions? Then your relationship may be affected by sleep quality issues.

While each of these problems represents a challenge to any relationship, there is at least one (but usually more than one) solution to each of these problems.

What is required?

Each of you needs to work together to identify what the problem is, generate a number of potential solutions, and then pick one to try. If the first solution does not seem effective, you go back either to brainstorming other solutions or to solutions you had brainstormed previously. Each and every one of these problems is solvable. All that is required is a desire on the part of each of you to make a commitment to generate potential solutions to improve peace and harmony in the bedroom.

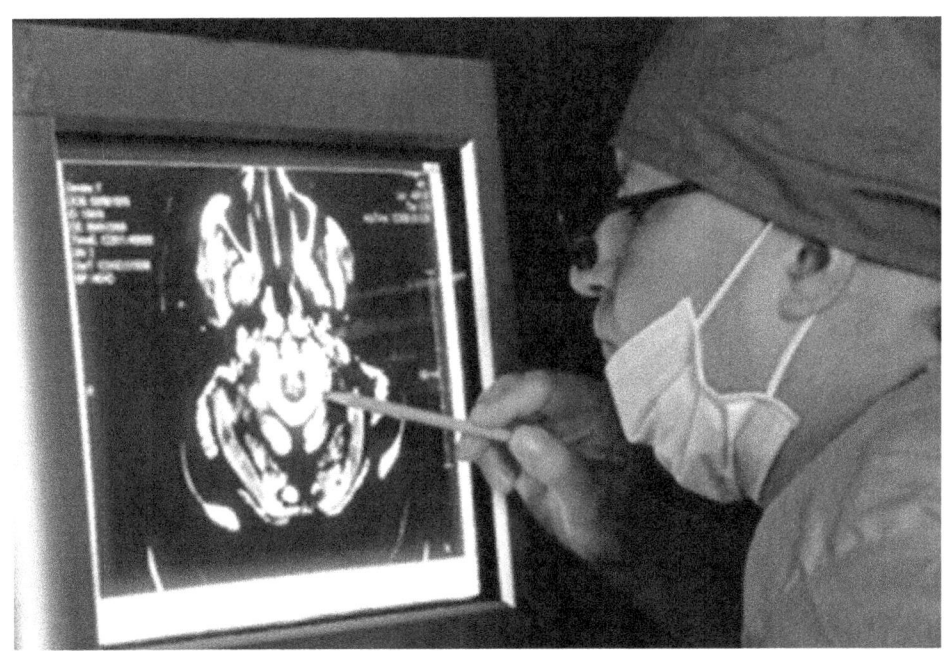

When Should You See a Doctor?

I f you believe that you cannot sleep because you are suffering from prolonged anxiety, depression, or a neurological disorder such as traumatic brain injury, Parkinson's disease, early dementia, etc., you should seek medical advice from your primary care provider (PCP). Your PCP may then suggest that you see a specialist in one of these noted areas.

Further, if you believe that you may have restless legs syndrome (irresistible urge to move your legs) or sleep apnea, a medical evaluation by a sleep medicine specialist is probably warranted. Ask yourself the following questions:

- Do you snore?
- Is your snoring loud?
- Do you snore more than three times per week?
- Does your snoring bother other people?
- Has anyone noticed that you stop breathing when you are sleeping?
- Are you overweight?
- Do you have high blood pressure?

If you answered yes to two or more of these questions, you may have sleep apnea or a sleep disorder that may require medical attention.

Sleep Medicine – What Is It?

According to the American Academy of Sleep Medicine (AASM)—a sleep medicine association for professionals dedicated to the treatment of sleep disorders such as sleep apnea and insomnia—accreditation is the gold standard by which the medical community and the public can evaluate sleep medicine services. The standards for accreditation established by the AASM ensure that sleep medicine providers display and maintain proficiency in areas such as testing procedures and policies, patient safety and follow-up, and provider and staff training.

To locate an accredited sleep medicine provider, you may wish to consider contacting the AASM. http://www.aasmnet.org/

What is Restless Legs Syndrome?

According to the Restless Legs Syndrome (RLS) Foundation, up to 10 percent of people living in win the Unites States have a mild form of RLS.

RLS is also known as Willis-Ekbom disease or WED. It is s neurological disease that affects 2 to 3 percent of the population. People with RLS or WED have an irresistible urge to move their legs. They feel that their legs are creeping, pulling, or tugging. Obviously, these uncomfortable feelings can cause significant problems with your ability to sleep and the quality of sleep that you experience.

There are medication and non-drug treatments for RLS. The FDA has approved Mirapex and Requip for the treatment of RLS. Non-drug treatments include taking some vitamin and mineral supplements, engaging in activities to distract oneself from the disorder, eliminating or avoiding medications that increase symptoms, and living a healthy lifestyle.

If you believe that you suffer from RLS, you should consult your healthcare provider as soon as possible. You will need a proper diagnosis and effective treatments to help you combat the effects of RLS and sleep better at night.

You may also wish to join the RLS Foundation. http://www.rls.org/

Are You Snoring?

Snoring may be a sign that that you are really suffering from sleep apnea. You should consult your healthcare provider to rule out sleep apnea through a thorough examination. However, sometimes snoring can be treated without significant medical intervention.

Getting Snoring Complaints? Try These Tips

With so many different things competing for your attention, the last thing you need is one more issue contriving to keep you from a full night of sleep. Unfortunately, snoring—your own or that of another person—often does just that. This section is packed with useful information to help you get the rest that you deserve.

To help reduce snoring, losing weight can be beneficial. People fail to realize that weight gain has an impact on breathing. By losing weight, you actually increase your air passage. Excessive weight impacts the comfort of your sleep. Losing weight is a basic way to help rid you of snoring and has many other health benefits.

Try a vapor rub just before bedtime to help alleviate snoring. These rubs are all natural and fairly reasonably priced and can continuously help you breathe better throughout the night, which will cut down on snoring. They are often successful at reducing snoring because they clear sinuses and regulate breathing.

If you or a loved one has noticed that you have a snoring problem, you should make an appointment to be evaluated in a sleep study. You may have sleep apnea, a condition where the esophagus closes and causes breathing problems such as snoring. If you have sleep apnea, you may be eligible for a c-pap machine that will create positive air flow while you sleep, curing snoring as well as breathing-related problems.

A great tip to help people reduce their snoring is to keep their room well ventilated. They should also keep cooler temperatures as both of these things have been shown to reduce the likelihood of snoring. If you don't have an air conditioner, simply prop open a window to keep your room cool.

Everyone likes to relax and enjoy luxury. If you have the means, get in a sauna as soon as you can before bed. The steam helps relieve congestion and also moisten your throat. If this isn't possible, consider purchasing a humidifier. When the air in your bedroom is dry, it can dehydrate the tissues and membranes of your nose and throat. This will irritate them, causing them to swell and restrict your airways which can cause you to snore. This can be exacerbated during the winter when heaters actively dry out the air in your home. If purchasing a humidifier is not an option, try taking a hot, steamy shower before bed to inhale some hydrating steam.

The side effects of some medications can cause dry or inflamed airways. The inflammations can cause mucus which can block airflow which, in turn, results in snoring. If you are currently taking medicine, find out if any of its side effects could be a cause of your snoring. If so, see if your doctor can suggest alternative medications without the side effects.

Tape your nose using specialized strips. Snoring is not only a problem in regard to your health, it can also impact the health of loved ones. When you are snoring so loudly that those near you can't get any sleep, it is a problem for everyone. Consider using un-medicated nasal strips to help control your snoring.

Avoid consuming dairy products, especially milk, before you go to bed. When you drink milk, it increases the production of mucus for some people. That mucus can build up in your throat and cause you to snore at night. If you wish to snore less, don't do dairy before bed.

There are many throat exercises out there that will help you strengthen your throat and stop snoring. One of these is to hold your mouth open, and then slide your jaw to the right. Hold it in place for thirty seconds. Then repeat by pushing your jaw to the left side and holding for thirty seconds. Stronger muscles mean less snoring.

If you smoke tobacco, you are more likely to snore when you sleep. The reason this occurs is that tobacco smoke contains irritants which can aggravate and constrict your airways, which results in snoring. Of course, for obvious other health reasons, it's best to just quit smoking.

Snoring can be a frustrating thing to deal with, but it may just be an underlying symptom of something larger, so make sure you are taking your overall health into consideration. If you are dealing with other health problems, speak with your doctor and find out if your snoring is actually being caused by something more serious, such as obesity or even smoking.

Avoid the consumption of alcohol before you go to bed in order to refrain from snoring. Because alcohol can relax the throat muscles, they may vibrate as air passes and cause snoring to occur. Allow several hours to pass after your last alcoholic beverage before you go to sleep to minimize or eliminate snoring.

Are you snoring a lot? Think about buying more pillows or simply purchasing a bigger one! Lying on your back tends to give you bad posture that will constrict the air passages within your throat. By raising your upper body while you sleep, the tissues in your throat will be more open and able to take in the airflow more easily.

With the advice and information from this section, hopefully there is more rest and relaxation in your future. Whether you have problems snoring or are forced to share a bed with someone who does, these helpful tips have come at just the right time. Before you lose another night of sleep, remember the information that you have just read.

Sleep Apnea Is a Serious Matter

If you've been diagnosed with sleep apnea, you may be in a state of confusion. Not knowing what to do is the hardest part of dealing with any affliction, so if you're looking for information, you've come to the right place. Keep reading for some of the best tips for dealing with sleep apnea.

This is an important topic so, if you believe you suffer from sleep apnea after reading this section, please consult a provider who is an expert in this area. According to the National Sleep foundation, obstructive sleep apnea (OSA) is also linked with depression.

In a study of 18,980 people in Europe conducted by Stanford researcher Maurice Ohayon, MD, PhD, people with depression were found to be five times more likely to suffer from sleep-disordered breathing. (OSA is the most common form of sleep-disordered breathing.) (17)

The good news is that treating OSA with continuous positive airway pressure (CPAP) may improve your mood considerably; a 2007 study of OSA patients who used CPAP for one year showed that improvements in complaints of depression were significant and lasting.

If you suffer from sleep apnea, try chewing on both sides of your mouth! It may sound odd, but if you think about it, chewing works all of your jaw muscles, so balanced strength and functionality may lessen the airway problems associated with sleep apnea. You might also try specific exercises that work all muscles in the jaw and throat.

You should let your employer or teachers know about your sleep apnea and give them more details about your symptoms. Feeling tired during the day will probably keep you from focusing and working efficiently—do not let your employer or teachers assume that you are not trying hard enough or that you're staying up late and partying.

If you decide to try a CPAP machine, give it at least a few weeks. A lot of sleep apnea patients give up before they really get a chance to get used to their machine. Wait until you are comfortable with sleeping while wearing a mask, and you should really notice a difference.

There are different kinds of masks you can use. Some masks cover your whole face while others cover only your nose and mouth. Try different products and choose one you feel comfortable wearing in bed. If you feel like your CPAP machine is not really working, try using a different mask with it.

To improve your sleep apnea, try losing weight. Several studies have shown that men who are overweight and have lost about 25 pounds within a year have seen drastic improvement in their symptoms. About 10 percent of those participants claimed that their sleep apnea went away and that they no longer needed treatment for it.

Invite your significant other to come with you to your next doctor's appointment. Not only will this educate your partner on sleep apnea, he or she can also inform your doctor about your condition through reporting on first-hand experiences. Your partner can, better than you, describe the patterns that occur while you sleep.

If your nasal airways are too narrow, try using nasal strips. You can buy these in any pharmacy, and they will not damage your airways like sprays do. Choose a quality product and apply the strips right before you go to bed. Breathing should be a little easier with these strips.

If you have sleep apnea, go to bed only when you are actually sleepy. You need to work to establish and maintain good sleep hygiene. This means that you when you get into bed, you actually fall asleep and stay asleep. Wait until you are actually sleepy before retiring for the night, and get back up if you have not fallen asleep within 20 minutes.

If you suffer from sleep apnea, it's important that you stay away from sleeping pills, cough syrup, or any other medication that may make you drowsy before going to sleep. These medications over-relax the throat muscles during sleep, even causing them to "collapse," making it hard for enough air to come through.

Get treated. Many people with sleep apnea do not even realize they have it. Snoring has become a fun joke, but it could be a sign of something more serious. If you find yourself feeling tired after sleeping, or if you have other symptoms that don't seem right, get medical treatment and find out if you have it.

Throat exercises will strengthen the muscles in the throat, keeping them from collapsing during the night. Try pressing your tongue against the roof of your mouth, and then hold it there for two or three minutes. You can also use a balloon. First, take a deep breath through your nasal passages, and then inflate the balloon as much as possible. Repeat this five times. These exercises will strengthen your airway muscles.

Your head and your throat should be aligned when you sleep. You can align your airways by sleeping on your side and propping your head with a small pillow. You should try different positions and wait a few minutes in each position to see which one allows you to breathe comfortably.

When suffering from severe sleep apnea, avoid driving or operating heavy machinery. Getting so little quality sleep drastically alters your ability to make quick, reflexive decisions, and you may easily fall asleep while driving, especially at night. Have someone else take over your driving duties until you can meet with your doctor to discuss treatment options.

While you may not be obese or even very overweight, even a couple of extra pounds can cause sleep apnea. That means even if you have a little belly, you should work to get rid of it and see if that removes your sleeping problems. You will thank yourself for it afterwards.

If you are always feeling drowsy during the day and find that it is hard to concentrate on the work you need to do, it may be time to speak to your doctor about the possibility of sleep apnea. You doctor can evaluate your symptoms and recommend some lifestyle changes that will help you get your sleep apnea under control.

Do not let your sleep apnea make you feel depressed. A lot of people have sleep apnea and are able to sleep peacefully thanks to their CPAP machine or mouth piece. You simply have to explore different options until you find something that works for you. In the meantime, deal as best as you can with the lack of sleep.

Now that you've reached the end of this section, you can see that there are things you can do about your sleep apnea. You don't have to simply accept it. Use what you've just learned to get a handle on this problem. You deserve to get the sleep that you need. But always consult your sleep professional before implementing any new method.

Back Pain: Tips for Some Welcome Relief and Better Sleep

Back pain can really affect your ability to sleep. (18) Your brain health will thank you if you can overcome back pain's interference with a good night's sleep. Pain gets in the way of every little thing you do and can really hamper your life and cramp your style. Whatever the cause of your back pain, there is relief. Read on for some fantastic tips and tricks to alleviate the problem of back pain in your life, starting now.

Make sure to avoid bending when you are standing or sitting to help avoid back pain. If you are standing, have your weight balanced on your feet. Using a chair designed to keep you sitting in a proper position can also do wonders for preventing issues with your back.

Make sure you stretch on a consistent basis if you are looking to reduce back pain! After every half hour of office work, take a few minutes to stretch. Make sure you stretch not only your back muscles but also your arms and shoulders! You'll find if you make this a consistent habit, your back pain is greatly relieved!

Avoid watching television in bed. We discussed elsewhere in this book the importance of avoiding other activities such as reading or watching TV in bed. But watching TV in bed can also contribute to pain in your back. Typically, people will prop themselves up in bed while enjoying some late-night television. These postures tend to be very bad and stressful for your back. So to decrease your back pain, contain your television activities to your living room and use your bedroom for what it was designed for!

Stretches and flexibility exercises can go a long way in preventing and even getting rid of back pain. If these stretches are done properly and according to guided direction, you will see positive results. Yoga is a good idea for certain situations, and especially for preventative measures. Yoga can also help with calming and relaxation before bedtime. Talk to your doctor, and do all that you can to prevent back pain.

You need to **pay close attention to your back when bending or kneeling.** If you feel any pulling, pain, or discomfort, stop immediately as these feelings signal strain on your back. If you stop immediately, you may be able to minimize any future potential issues and discomfort with your back.

Gentle compression can help with back pain, reducing its impact on sleep onset. A compression pack applied to the injured area provides some level of support and comfort. It can let your body move easier and make you feel a bit more comfortable. A simple, large elastic strap, wrapped loosely, is a good choice for a compression pack. Avoid wrapping it too tightly or discomfort could result.

If you are suffering from back pain, **look into acupuncture as a possible treatment.** More and more medical practitioners are using this method to treat patients effectively. Upon insertion, the needles stimulate specific nerves that trigger the brain and spinal cord to release chemicals that can help to reduce pain. Many back pain sufferers have found relief using this method.

If you have back pain, **take a look at your mattress.** If your mattress is very old, it likely is not supporting your back properly, and you could potentially be causing damage to your spine every time you are asleep. So, if your mattress is very lumpy, soft, or saggy, consider buying a new one to save your back.

If your back is stiff in the morning, it may help to spend some time stretching before you even get out of bed. While asleep, blood leaves the back to go to organ groups, which means that if you wake up and try to move right away, your back muscles won't be ready.

Many people do not know this, but **nicotine hinders the flow of nutrient-rich blood to spinal discs.** This easily causes back pain and therefore means smokers are highly susceptible to back pain. If you smoke, it is recommended you should quit for many reasons, and now you can make this yet another reason.

If you have noticed that you keep getting back pain during the day, you need to figure out what is causing this in order to fix it. When you think you know what is causing the pain, make sure to change that behavior or action, and check to see if your pain lessens.

Taking a long, brisk walk can help to loosen up your muscles and eliminate the back pain you're dealing with. We have discussed elsewhere the value of exercise to sleep in general and brain health in particular. Remember to exercise earlier in the day and at least three hours before bedtime.

While walking might not actually cure the pain permanently, the exercise will help soothe the pain by stretching the muscles and keeping them warm. Take the dog around the block or walk to the store and back.

Losing weight can help you with your back pain. While the definition of "overweight" is open to a lot of interpretation, there is a definite limit to the amount of weight your back and spine are meant to carry. If you go beyond this weight, you place undue strain on your back every day. Cutting unnecessary pounds can free you from this source of back pain.

If you are sitting in a chair working at a desk, **make sure your chair has good support** and is the right height. You should never have to strain to get on or off a chair. If you are not comfortable, any office supply store will carry a variety of chairs.

Make sure to always remember to stretch before you attempt any sort of exercise or physical activity. Stretching allows your back to get prepared for the activity to come. Forgetting this important step can lead to serious pain later on, which is what we want to avoid.

Rest your back if you are experiencing back pain. If you do not give your back a rest when it needs it, you are potentially causing permanent injury to your joints, ligaments, tendons, and muscles. Do not underestimate the healing power of giving your aching back a well-deserved rest.

To properly treat back pain and swelling with ice and avoid damaging sensitive skin, be sure to use care when applying the ice. Avoid applying ice directly to the skin. To create your own ice pack, use ice cubes or chips wrapped in a soft, dampened towel. Apply the ice pack to the injured area for no longer than 15 minutes.

Hopefully you have found some very practical advice on how to reduce the amount of pain your back gives you in your day-to-day life. Put the tips and tricks from this segment into practice beginning today and reduce the aches and pains in your back as soon as tomorrow. Your brain will thank you and you will surely sleep better tonight.

Do You Still Smoke?

Our discussion of brain health and sleep would be incomplete if we didn't at least touch on this topic. Nicotine is a stimulant and thus causes arousal which can affect the quality of sleep. Cigarette smokers were significantly more likely than nonsmokers to report problems going to sleep, problems staying asleep, daytime sleepiness, minor accidents, depression, and high daily caffeine intake. (19)

Consider the following tips to help you get moving in the right direction if you use nicotine and have decided to stop. Quitting smoking is one of the best choices you can make for your health. Smoking affects you negatively in a variety of ways. The following segment will give you some tips to help you make your decision to quit a lasting one.

To improve your odds of quitting smoking for good, **don't combine your effort to quit with another goal, particularly weight loss.** You already have enough stress and cravings to deal with just trying to quit smoking. If you try to wean yourself from something else at the same time, you are likely to fail at both.

Throw away your cigarettes and lighters. This will make it impossible to smoke unless you leave the house. It serves to remind you how much of a hassle it is to smoke and leaves you without any. When you do this, keep yourself busy with other activities so that you don't think about smoking.

Once you quit smoking, have regular celebrations. After you go two weeks without smoking, treat yourself to a movie. Once you go a month, eat at a fancy restaurant. Once you go six months, purchase some item that you've been wanting. Once you go an entire year without smoking, have a party for yourself. Invite all your friends and family to celebrate this milestone. These little celebrations can assist you in kicking this bad habit to the curb so that you can enjoy a healthier life.

To help you quit smoking, some people say that eating low-calorie snack foods is very effective. Try purchasing mini carrots, cut-up broccoli, cauliflower, dried fruit, low-calorie cereal, or sugar-free candy. Consuming any of these items when you have the desire to smoke can help control cravings and keep your mouth busy.

Whenever you get the urge smoke, try exercising. As mentioned elsewhere in this book, exercise is great for brain health in general and sleep in particular. Physical exercise can also be a great diversion in place of smoking, apart from being optimal for the body and one's conventional good health. Small, concise blasts of exercise will help conquer those sudden cravings that come from nowhere. So try exercise to quit smoking!

Don't assume that a nicotine-withdrawal medication has to have nicotine in it. While it is true that you can find an alternate source of nicotine and reduce your levels of it, you could just try a prescription medication that blocks your need for nicotine. Consult your physician about a medicine that might just kill your cravings.

Think specifically about how quitting smoking will improve your life and your sleep. Think of all the health conditions you can worry less about. Think about how much money you can save. Think about how the whiteness of your teeth and the smell of your home will improve. Most importantly, think of how much less likely your children will be to smoke.

Put aside the money you would have normally spent on cigarettes, and save it for something that you really want, like a new outfit, some nice furniture, or a weekend away. Not only will you be feeling healthier, but you'll soon see how much money you can save now that you're not smoking.

To help yourself stay quit, **spend time in places where you cannot smoke.** Go to the movies, a museum, a nice restaurant, a coffee shop, or the library. The pleasant surroundings will be a nice distraction from cravings, and knowing that you can't smoke in the first place will make you less likely to want one.

The best way to quit for good is to quit for the right reasons. You should not quit for the people around you. **You should quit for**

yourself. You should make a decision that you want to live a happier, healthier lifestyle and stick to it. This is the best way to ensure success.

If you are a smoker who lights up more in social situations, you should plan ways to avoid joining your friends for a cigarette when you are socializing. While dining, stay at the table if your friends go outside to smoke. If you're at a party and people are smoking, find a non-smoker to chat with. Finding ways to not be around smokers will make it easier for you to quit.

Become a secondhand smoker. After you make it three weeks and have made tobacco freedom your new habit, you will still have cravings from time to time. You might not want to smoke, but you just miss the lovely smell. You can stand downwind of current smokers for a brief moment of nostalgic aroma and then move on. If it is distasteful to you (and it probably will be), you are well on your way to permanently eliminating the addiction.

You should make sure you have an appropriate reward system in place for such a difficult task. You will want to reward yourself for at least the first three days of quitting and the first two weeks. After that, monthly milestones are worth a celebration until you hit the annual mark. You can choose your reward based on the time elapsed as well, making success that much sweeter.

Quit smoking with a buddy. Having someone else with whom to commiserate and celebrate will make your success even sweeter. Choose a friend, relative, or co-worker who also wants to quit, or pair up with someone on an online support forum. Having someone by your side will make the process much easier to tolerate and will help you stay accountable.

Write down why you're quitting ahead of time and keep that list handy. When that craving hits you, refer to your list for motivation. Understanding ahead of time why quitting is important to you will help to keep you focused in those moments of weakness, and it might even help to get you back on track if you should slip up.

If the cigarettes you smoke after meals are some of the hardest to give up, replace the habit of smoking after eating with brushing your teeth or chewing minty gum. Slowly, you will break your old habit and build a much healthier association between finishing a meal and also freshening your breath.

For most of us, quitting smoking is not easy. The addiction to nicotine is a powerful one and overcoming it takes much determination. Do not be discouraged if you are not successful the first time. The most important thing is that you continue on your path to quitting. Your brain, heart, lungs, and your sleep will thank you. Good luck!

What about Medication for Sleep?

Going to the local Food Mart off base was a common practice for Sgt. Oliver (not his real name). But when Oliver awoke one night to find himself in the parking lot of the Food Mart, he was shocked and frightened. How did he get there? More importantly, how did he get there without killing himself or someone else?

After reviewing his current medications, it became apparent that Sgt. Oliver needed to have his medications reconciled by the pharmacologist on the team. We soon determined that Sgt. Oliver was getting up during the night and "sleep driving." This is an occurrence known as "complex sleep-related behavior." Other behaviors include having sex, eating, making phone calls, and, of course, driving while not fully awake. The frightening part about complex sleep-related behavior is that most people don't remember these events later. In other words, they have amnesia.

Complex behaviors like these are a potential side effect of sedative-hypnotic products—a class of medications used to help people suffering from insomnia fall asleep and stay asleep. (20)

It should be obvious to the reader that complex behaviors, such as sleep driving, are potentially dangerous to the insomniac as well as others in the community. Commonly prescribed medications for sleep are known to have this effect on people, and it may not be as rare as some might suggest.

Regardless of the impact, what is clear is that medications used to induce and maintain sleep have always been intended for short-term use. For example, sleep medications are sometimes used to help those who have lost a loved one, are in bereavement, or are in the midst of a short-term hospitalization.

Here is a direct quote from a drug insert for a hypnotic (sleep medication): "X should normally be taken for short periods of time. If you take X for 2 weeks or longer, X may not help you sleep as well as it did when you first began to take the medication. If you take X for a long time, you also may develop dependence ('addiction,' a need to continue taking the medication) on X."

The description of the medication from the National Institutes of Health website continues as follows: "Do not stop taking X without talking to your doctor, especially if you have taken it for longer than 2 weeks. If you suddenly stop taking X, you may develop unpleasant feelings or mood changes or you may experience other withdrawal symptoms such as shakiness, lightheadedness, stomach and muscle cramps, nausea, vomiting, sweating, flushing, tiredness, uncontrollable crying, nervousness, panic attack, difficulty falling asleep or staying asleep, uncontrollable shaking of a part of your body, and rarely, seizures."

Now don't misunderstand me, sleep medication can be helpful. But the sad fact is that many people who start down that road don't stop. After a time, these sleep medications require higher doses to have the same effect, or they simply stop working altogether.

What about allergic reactions to sleep medications? Well, other rare but potential side effects of sedative-hypnotic sleep medications include trouble breathing and severe facial swelling, which can occur as early as the first time the drug is taken.

Basically, severe allergic reactions can affect a person's ability to breathe, can affect other body systems as well, and can even be fatal at times. Although many allergic reactions are probably very rare, people should be aware that they can occur. You need to communicate well with your pharmacist and prescribing doctor. Why? Simply put, because these adverse reactions may be difficult to notice when you are falling asleep.

Sleep Aids Bought without a Prescription

Not all medications for sleep require a prescription, but that doesn't mean that you don't have to be cautious. The FDA has approved over-the-counter (OTC) medications for use up to two weeks to help relieve occasional sleeplessness in people ages 12 and older. You should clearly see your doctor if you continue to have sleeping problems beyond two weeks. Remember, as we have discussed elsewhere in this book, sleep problems may have numerous causes and should be properly diagnosed.

Generally, OTC sleep aids are non-habit forming. Further, they generally do not present the risk of allergic reactions and complex sleep-related behaviors that are known to occur with sedative-hypnotic drugs.

However, just because they're available without a prescription doesn't mean they don't have side effects. Because they don't have the same level of precision as prescription drugs, people feel drowsy for longer than eight hours after taking them. Thus, you may wake up feeling groggy or have trouble waking up on time for work or school.

It is important to remember that prescription and nonprescription medications can affect people differently. They are not for all of us. You should always read the label and precautions carefully. Use caution when taking any medication and always consult with your medical provider.

How Can I Sleep Better for Mental and Physical Health?

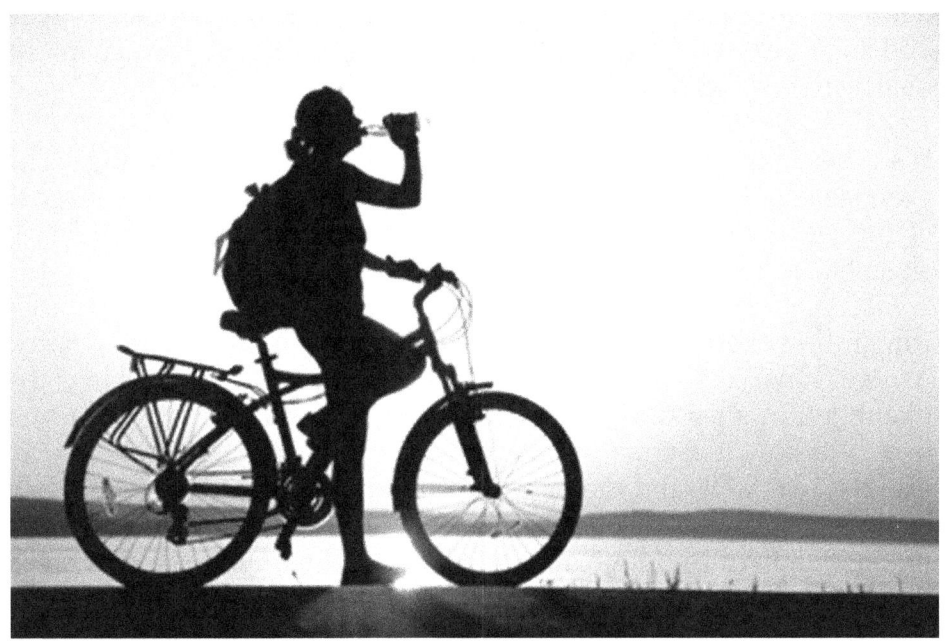

Fitness and Sleep

Exercise is important for cardiovascular and brain health, but did you know that being fit can help you sleep better tonight? It's true and we will discuss some tips on how to get started.

People who are more physically fit have higher levels of slow-wave sleep (SWS) than unfit people. Second, following exercise, the level of SWS increased in fit individuals but remained unchanged in unfit subjects. (21)

Getting exercise and keeping physically fit within the context of your age and medical status is vital to getting a good night's sleep. Get guidance from your doctor if you have health challenges that need to be accommodated in your fitness program.

I am writing this particular section of the book on a beautiful Saturday afternoon in southwest Georgia. I decided to take a break and take our yellow Labrador retriever, Bambi, for a walk in the nearby fields and through the woods.

It's a beautiful 75 degrees and there's a light breeze blowing. The exercise is helping to refresh me. While that was really the purpose of the walk, the advantage of this walk will, in fact, be that I will sleep better tonight.

Integrating exercise into your daily life is important to sleep quality. As we have discussed elsewhere in this book, increasing the likelihood of a good night's sleep does not begin when you get into bed. Rather, it begins earlier in the day as you make choices to exercise, eat well, and manage your daily stress. As your sleep debt begins to grow as the day progresses, the choices that you have made earlier in the day will contribute to the quality of your sleep that night.

Let's discuss some of the important factors related to **fitness. Exercising and fitness do not have to be difficult.** There are simple methods anyone can utilize to get into better physical shape.

When you take time to apply a proper fitness routine, it really does show. It shows that you care about taking care of yourself and your health and that you are trying to look the best that you can. That is admirable. As with anything else, you can always improve. The following are some tips to help.

Workouts can be very hard to finish, especially if you do not enjoy going to the gym. The best thing that you can do is find extra motivation and incentive to get to where you want to be. Think of all the people who said you could not get skinny and use that to fuel your fire in the gym.

If you have hired a coach or trainer, pay your fitness trainer in advance. This makes you much more likely to follow through on your workout because most trainers do not give refunds. Paying them in advance will likely give you a heads up on the other clients as well because your trainer will pay more attention to you.

To increase your level of motivation, go to the gym with a friend. Tell them all about the goals that you are trying to achieve so that they can help and motivate you to get where you want to be. Positive encouragement can go a long way in achieving top results.

In order to get the most out of your weightlifting sessions and gain as much muscle as possible, it is important to eat plenty of protein. Eating four to eight ounces of protein every single day is a great way to get all of the protein that your body needs and will also help to boost testosterone levels. Studies have proven that meat eaters gain muscle more easily than vegetarians.

Try to devise a healthy eating plan and diet for yourself in addition to your workout regimen. The healthier you eat, the easier it is to get into shape. You should also notice that you have more energy when you work out when you eat healthier as well. Remember you are what you eat and your body reacts to what you put into it.

Scheduling your exercise routines in the early morning can provide some additional fitness benefits beyond the immediate value of working out. When you get your exercise done first thing, you will experience increased energy levels throughout the rest of the day. You will also have the powerful psychological boost that comes from knowing you have already met the day's fitness goals.

Remember that it is important that you not exercise within three hours of bedtime. Exercise will increase your energy as previously noted. We need you to be winding down with a relaxation routine as your bedtime approaches.

Exercising with your dog like I do can be a great motivator. Having to take your dog out can increase the frequency of your workouts as well as your enjoyment of them. Some health clubs even offer classes or activities that can be done with your pet, such as "doggy yoga"!

Fitness can be a very enjoyable activity. However, for a beginner, the special gear and equipment used for some of the routines can be downright intimidating. So, what should a novice do to learn how to use them? Well, read the following tips, of course!

Getting in shape, which helps you sleep better, doesn't mean that you have to be miserable. If you find an activity that you actually enjoy, it will help the time pass faster as you start to get in shape. Additionally, this will help you stay motivated on the days you really don't want to go to the gym.

Walking: We do it every day, but there's a good chance that we could be doing it a lot more. Even minor adjustments in your daily number of steps can contribute to weight loss. Try parking at the end of the lot, taking the stairs instead of the elevator, or simply taking a leisurely stroll around the block.

Sometimes it can be hard to maintain a daily exercise regimen, but **here are a few quick tips to help you stick with it.**

1. Set a daily alarm or daily reminder on your phone to encourage you to exercise, and make it encouraging and positive. Remember, this is something you want to do!
2. Set the reminder for a time when you usually don't have anything pressing to do, such as after you come home from work or right when you wake up or go to bed.
3. Remember, you can split your daily exercise into two 15-minute sessions. It can sometimes be easier to find 15 minutes than it can be to find 30, so perhaps set two alarms during the day.

Be sure to keep a regular schedule to maintain optimum energy and optimum fitness. **Go to sleep and get up at the same time daily**—even if it is an upside-down schedule that has you sleeping during the day and working at night. If you fall off your schedule, fast for a day and go to bed at your regular hour to reset your internal clock.

You can easily save your back from injury when lifting weights by squeezing your butt cheeks together tightly. This causes your posture to improve while lifting because it stabilizes your spine. This stabilization protects your back from strain or injury, so try doing this during your next weight-lifting session.

If you feel like you're in a rut, try something new. Try a different workout or a different program. Your boredom may be the result of the methods you are trying and you might just need something new. Switch up your fitness routines and you might discover something new that you enjoy.

Keep a good pace! Reciting the alphabet can get you on your way to being in great physical shape. How? A simple way to know if you are exercising at the correct pace is to say the letters out loud: if you cannot say them without puffing, you are working too hard! Working too hard can lead to strain.

A good tip for people who are looking to get back into shape is to forget about what other people think. Oftentimes, people are self-conscious about their bodies, but you should recognize that everyone in the gym is trying to look better just like you are, so relax.

When working out, you should not stress about fixed rest periods between each set. **You should rest whenever you need.** Typically, this will be less in the early sets because your body is fresh. As you become fatigued, make your rest periods longer. If you do this, you can potentially cut your workout time by around 15 to 20 percent.

To get immediate results from your workout routine, **try doing circuit training.** This technique involves a series of rapid moves between different exercises with no rest break in between. You might go from squats to pushups to jumping jacks. Circuit training lets you burn fat while strengthening your muscles, so you get faster results.

Never let fear stand in the way when trying to reach a fitness goal. It is normal to feel a little unsure of yourself if you are doing something new. You will have a lot to learn, so just remember that once you go at it consistently, you will get more comfortable and make progress.

A great fitness tip for runners who experience sore calves would be to sleep on your belly and let your feet dangle off the bed. Over the course of the night, your calves will stretch out from being in this position. Of course, stretching, warming up, and cooling down are also going to assist you with this.

If you are just starting out on the road to healthy living, avoid overdoing your exercising. Do not try to work out too vigorously. If you do, it will reduce your energy and may cause injury. Any exercise is an improvement to not exercising. So if you can only work out for 10 minutes, it is better than 10 minutes of not exercising.

Now you should be able to see why fitness can be such an enjoyable activity to participate in. If you are more fit and exercise regularly, you will sleep better tonight. Your brain will thank you. There is so much fun and many benefits to be had as you try to get yourself in better shape. With these tips in mind, you can start a better fitness routine and sleep better tonight.

Does Nutrition Affect Sleep and Memory?

Eating right and following a good nutritional plan is important for the health and welfare of your mind, body, and soul. (22) With so much advice from so many so-called experts out there, it can be hard to make good choices. The advice in this section stands apart from the rest. So, if you heed it, you will be on right path.

The general rule of thumb was that you should avoid caffeine approximately three or four hours before bedtime. Recent sleep research has increased that to 10 hours before bedtime. Thus, avoid caffeine-containing beverages such as coffee, soda, tea, and energy drinks before bedtime. You should also avoid caffeine-containing foods, such as chocolate, or over-the-counter medications that might contain caffeine. Following these suggestions will give you the best opportunity to get to sleep at the time you determine.

If you're pregnant, check with your doctor about getting a magnesium prescription. Magnesium deficiency can lead to cramps, premature delivery, or even a miscarriage. It's recommended that you take in at least 310 milligrams of magnesium every day. Your

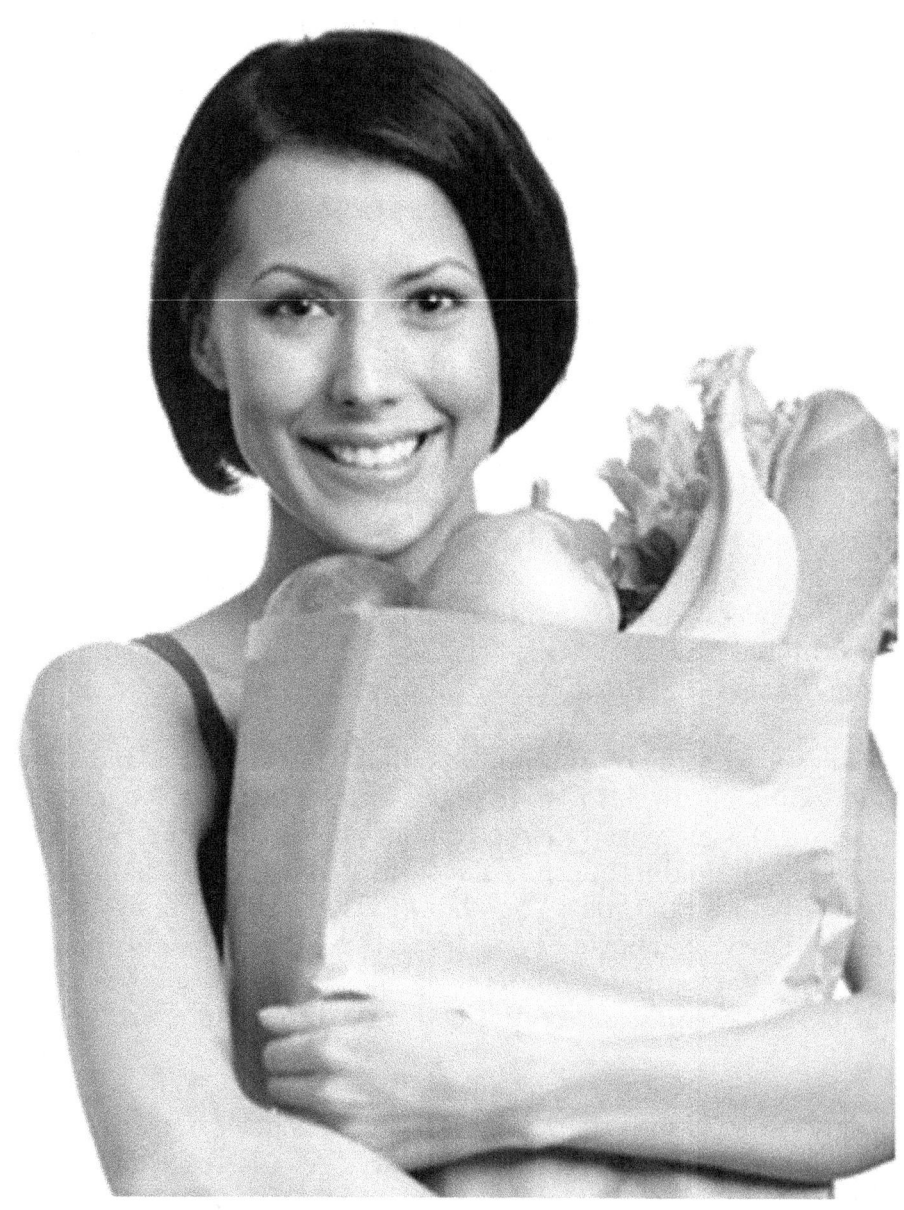

doctor may be able to write you a prescription for a daily dose of magnesium.

Make sure that you know the difference between simple and complex carbohydrates because eating the wrong ones can make you gain weight while the other can help you lose. Eating complex carbohydrates like brown rice and whole grain bread help keep you full for much longer so that you will end up eating less.

Avoid eating too many carbohydrates at midday as you will be more likely to feel tired and to want to take a nap. Daytime napping should generally be avoided in order to sleep through the night and increase the length of nighttime sleep.

Conversely, some complex carbohydrates later in the day may actually cause drowsiness and aid in sleep onset. However, don't overdo the carbohydrates.

A healthy diet with good nutrition is, almost always, a varied diet. While the human body can derive adequate nutrition from constant ingestion of a few foods, the human mind rebels at the prospect. Adding many healthy alternatives into a diet keeps it exciting and novel. A varied diet is an easier diet to stick to.

Riboflavin is a great energy booster and supplement to add to your arsenal when you wake up. If you have a lot of energy, your body processes flow very smoothly, and the chance of toxins building up internally is very slim. Riboflavin also halts the formation of acne and creates a beautiful radiance to your face.

Always make breakfast a part of your day. Your body has gone without fuel for the entire night, and skipping breakfast is like pressing down the gas pedal on a car with an empty gas tank. Many people think that by skipping breakfast they will save calories. However, studies have shown that eating breakfast gets your metabolism going, prevents you from overeating later on in the day, and ultimately helps you lose weight. To maximize your results, choose protein and fiber-rich foods over sugary doughnuts. Those sugary foods will cause you to feel like napping.

Color is a key factor in choosing vegetables for good nutrition—the darker the color the better. Vitamin A can be found in yellow, orange, and dark green vegetables, such as pumpkin, peppers, carrots, and spinach. The nutrition found in these delicious vegetables can boost your immune system's functioning by neutralizing the free radicals that attack healthy cells.

Eating unsaturated fats is generally preferable to saturated fats. Saturated fats are known to have a negative effect on the human body's arteries because of their tendency to accumulate in them. These platelets of cholesterol can slowly build up and eventually block passages. Obviously, this could impact brain health over time. Unsaturated fats are unable to perform the same procedure because they lack the small shape of saturated fats.

Vitamins play a very important role in our life. Some of them can be synthesized by our body, but most of them should be included in our daily food. It is a good practice to eat lots of fresh fruits, vegetables, soy, whole grain bakery products, nuts, and beans. Without these building blocks we become sick.

When considering a diet that provides an adequate nutrition level, be sure to include low-fat milk. Milk provides many nutrients—including calcium and protein—that the body needs. Studies have shown that drinking milk does benefit muscle growth and also the body's ability to maintain a healthy body-fat content.

Portion out your foods. Measuring the actual amount of food you are eating can help you prevent overeating. One easy way to get the proper amount is to use a measuring cup as a serving spoon. Doing this makes you more aware of what you are actually scooping onto your plate.

Try new ways to eat foods you eat on a regular basis. Instead of just eating plain yogurt, pour a bit of honey in and experience a new taste sensation. Instead of always steaming broccoli, you may want to try frying it up with a few other vegetables. You'll be more likely to eat healthily if you have fun with it.

So many of the foods we eat today are filled with preservatives and artificial ingredients that are addictive and not good for your body. Stay away from buying any type of canned food or food that comes from a box. Make your own meals at home so that you know exactly what you are eating.

The following are some foods that have been associated with both good nutrition and that promote calmness for a good night's sleep. Foods that contain tryptophan, which is a natural amino acid, can assist you in getting to sleep easier. There is some evidence that tryptophan may also help you sleep longer. Tryptophan is utilized by the body and brain to produce melatonin and serotonin, two substances that cause you to sleep.

The following foods are highest in tryptophan:

- Whole grains
- Various nuts such as peanuts, soybean nuts, and hazelnuts
- Turkey (remember those naps after Thanksgiving dinner?)
- Tuna, clams, and oysters
- Soft cheeses, cottage cheese, and milk or yogurt
- Chickpeas and lentils
- Brown rice, hummus, and beans
- Eggs
- Sunflower and sesame seeds

So, in order to keep your brain, body, and sleep on the right path, you need to establish good nutrition as a foundation in your life. This can be achieved by learning about nutrition and taking the advice offered here.

Can Journaling Help?

What is journaling and how may it help you sleep more effectively? You recall that stress is your enemy with regard to sleep. Consequently, a good way of handling stress is to be able to express your thoughts, feelings, and attitudes through journaling.

Journaling is really a stress-management tool. Through self-discovery and exploration you are able to learn more effectively what patterns of thought processes and emotional concerns you may be experiencing that are actually interfering with your ability to sleep at night.

Simply put, journaling is a way for you to identify thoughts and feelings so that you are more effectively able to deal with them in a way that will prevent them from interfering with your sleep at night.

Research has indicated that journaling can help people improve their overall cognitive efficiency. (23) It can also strengthen your ability to counteract the negative effects of stress. Therapists have found journaling to be an effective tool to help people manage severe forms of stress. Through journaling they are able to identify certain thoughts and feelings which they then can clarify with a therapist. This really is not our purpose, however.

Some people prefer to use a computer word processor to journal, but a pen or pencil will work just as well. Set aside approximately 10 or 15 minutes a day for journaling. Allow yourself to express your thoughts and feelings about the things that are happening in your life.

Once you've gotten the hang of journaling, you then may be able to identify certain patterns of thoughts and feelings which are actually causing you to experience stress. By identifying the stressors, you will be much better able to use a Worry Method discussed elsewhere in the book to effectively identify potential solutions to your concerns.

If you've never done journaling before, it may be fun to give it a try. Consider doing it for at least two weeks. You will be amazed at what you are able to discover about your thought processes and feelings.

What about Nightmares?

What is a nightmare? A nightmare is a dream state in which the person experiences visual sequences that often depict situations that are disturbing or frightening to the individual. If nightmares occur frequently, they are considered to be a sleep disorder.

Nightmares generally occur during rapid-eye-movement sleep or in the deeper stages of sleep known as stage III and IV. Nightmares often lead to feelings of anxiety. According to the American Sleep Association (ASA), nightmares are very common and occur in up to 80–90 percent of people at some point in their lives.

Children as young as three can experience nightmares. However, it is generally the case that nightmares decrease over time. Nevertheless, it is common for adults to have nightmares from time to time. Nightmares could reflect a more serious problem, including posttraumatic stress disorder (PTSD) or other significant, unresolved internal conflicts.

According to the ASA, **chronic nightmares** which result in a sleep disorder occur in approximately only 5 percent of the population. Nightmares are not something that you can treat on your own.

If you belong to the 5 percent of people who are experiencing nightmares, it is important for you to discuss this with your personal care physician. He or she will then refer you to a sleep medicine specialist and/or a clinical psychologist who is skilled in helping people overcome the internal conflicts and circumstances that may be leading to the recurrent and frequent nightmare problem.

Because deep sleep is extremely important to overall health, it is important that the nightmares be resolved. If you were to take medication that would prevent deeper sleep to avoid nightmares, it would have other negative consequences to your health as we discussed elsewhere in this book. It is important that you get deep sleep in order to consolidate memories and maintain good health.

A promising new therapy has emerged in recent years. In a randomized controlled trial involving 168 participants reported by Kraków in 2001 in the Journal of the American Medical Association, nightmare frequency reduced significantly with treatment at three- and six-month follow-up. (24) In other words, the treatment effects lasted.

Imagery rehearsal therapy is a brief, very well-tolerated treatment that appears to decrease chronic nightmares. The therapy also improves sleep quality and has been known to decrease symptoms of posttraumatic stress disorder in both military veterans and victims of sexual assault.

Sleep Restriction: An Effective Approach

Each and every one of the things that we have discussed throughout this book is important to improving sleep quality and maintaining good brain health. For each individual a particular method or technique or strategy or problem area is significant for them.

Most often in my experience in working with people with sleep problems over the years, including the past two and half years we have been working with active-duty soldiers, more than one method is often required to overcome sleep difficulties.

One of the most effective approaches I have found in reducing chronic insomnia is sleep restriction. (3) Sleep restriction is a method that requires you to become acutely aware of the hours that you spend in bed versus the hours you spend in bed sleeping. Consequently, it's extremely important that you keep the sleep log weekly. The following is an example of the sleep log that I have found to be helpful for many people:

Sleep Log

Day of the Week	Monday	
Date	11/1	
Total Nap Time	50 minutes	
Time in Bed	11 p.m.	
In-Bed Time before Sleep Onset	45 minutes	
Total Time Awake from Sleep Interruptions	60 minutes	
Wake-Up Time	7 a.m.	

Out-of-Bed Time	7:30 a.m.	
Total Sleep Time	315 minutes	
Time In Bed	480 minutes	

Total Sleep Time = Time in Bed – Time Awake

In this example, the person went to bed at 11 p.m. and got out of bed at 7:30 a.m. Thus, they were in bed for a total of 8.5 hours.

However, they napped for 50 minutes; they were in bed before sleep started for 45 minutes; they were awake a total of 60 minutes for interruptions; they lay in bed for 30 minutes in the morning before getting out of bed at 7:30 a.m.

Thus, we add 50 + 45 + 60 + 30 = 185 minutes in bed not sleeping. So, while they were in bed 480 minutes, they were sleeping only 315 minutes. Therefore, going forward we would restrict the time in bed to 315 minutes + 30 minutes or 345 minutes.

We then set the bedtime based upon the time they must get up in the morning. If the awakening time remains 7:30 a.m., we will set the new bedtime as 1:45 a.m.

As our sample person begins to sleep more continuously through the night, we will back up the bedtime 30 to 45 minutes. Our goal is approximately seven hours of quality, uninterrupted or only briefly interrupted sleep.

Sleep restriction therapy is based upon Spielman's work in 1983. When sleep opportunity exceeds sleep ability, wakefulness is a result and sleep is much less efficient. By restricting time in bed there is an increase in sleep efficiency which is enhanced by using sleep deprivation as a tool.

Let's review these instructions: First, you need to determine your average sleep time with the sleep log. Specifically this refers to your sleep ability. You will then want to limit your time in bed (or your sleep opportunity) to the average sleep time. You will start with the desired wake-up time and count backwards. Five hours time in bed is a minimum for most people. You can actually plan activities to fill extra time. Once you have done a sleep log, you should reevaluate it once per week. If your sleep efficiency is greater than 85 or 90 percent, you can increase the time in bed by 15 to 30 minutes. Otherwise you should maintain the current schedule. If your sleep efficiency drops below 80 percent, you can reduce your time in bed by 15 or 30 minutes. Generally it takes approximately four to six weeks for most people to show improved sleep quality.

Sleep restriction can be difficult to follow for some people. It's important that you understand that sleep deprivation may cause you to be even drowsier during the daytime. Therefore, when operating machinery or driving a motor vehicle, you need to be particularly careful. We do not use sleep restriction with patients who have epilepsy.

As we discussed elsewhere, it is very common for people to be engaging in activities other than sleep while in bed. We have discussed how these activities are generally not appropriate. If you are sleeping well, you are able to get to sleep within 15 minutes of the time that you get into bed. You may spend another 15 minutes in the morning rousing yourself before you get out of bed. This would be considered to be a normal sleep-habit pattern.

Let's discuss an example: John needs to get out of bed at 7 a.m. He is kept a sleep schedule during the past week and has discovered that he is averaging five hours of sleep per night. He determined this after deducting the amount of time he lay in bed without sleeping, the number of sleep interruptions he had during the night, and the amount of time that he stayed in bed in the morning.

Because John awakens at 7 a.m., he must subtract five hours from 7 a.m. to determine his bedtime. He will also subtract 30 minutes. Thus, his bedtime now becomes 1:30 a.m. All this may seem strange to you at first, but you need to realize that John has been spending a considerable amount of time awake in bed. His typical bedtime would either be 10:30 or 11:00 p.m. This would accommodate him getting at least seven to eight hours of sleep with a half hour added for being awake a brief period of time prior to going to sleep and the 15 minutes in the morning.

John implements this sleep schedule. He is very tired for the first several days. However, he has noted that he is sleeping through the night with perhaps one exception of a rising to go to bathroom. Thereafter he returns to sleep quickly. Because he continues to be very tired in the morning, it is time for us to back up the sleep schedule. We now take another half hour to 45 minutes from the time that he was originally going to bed at 1:30 and now have him go to bed at a proximally 12:15. We continue to back up this sleep schedule until we reach his desired time of 10:30 or 11:00 p.m. to go to sleep. This is sleep restriction.

In approximately four to five weeks, John is now sleeping seven and a half hours each night. His sleep is rarely interrupted, and, if it is, he is able to return to sleep rather quickly. John has also implemented taking a bath before bedtime which relaxes him, increases his core body temperature, and causes him to feel drowsy as he gets into bed. He also cut out caffeine earlier in the day. He now does not drink caffeine after approximately 11 a.m. He started walking five times a week. He walks for approximately 20 minutes at lunch time and frequently walks for about 30 minutes to 45 minutes after work. John has implemented some of the strategies that he has learned through reading this book. He is now sleeping better and has improved his ability to concentrate and focus during the day. John has improved his memory and brain health.

Sleep Better Now Instructions

1. **Sleep only as much as needed to feel refreshed the following day.**
   Definitive time in bed helps consolidate and deepen sleep. Spending exaggerated time in bed can lead to fragmented and shallow sleep.

2. **Have a standard wake-up time, seven days a week.**
   A standard wake-up time in the morning will help set your "biological clock" and lead to a regular sleep ending.

3. **Your bedroom should be cheerful and free from light and noise.**
   A comfortable bed and bedroom environment will reduce the likelihood that you will wake up during the night. Exceptionally warm or cold rooms can disrupt sleep as well. A quiet environment promotes sleep better than a noisy one. Noises can be masked with background white noise (such as the noise of a fan) or with earplugs. Bedrooms may be darkened with black-out shades or even sleep masks can be worn. Position clocks out of sight because clock-watching can increase worry about lack of sleep.

4. **Refrain or Stay Away from Caffeine 6 Hours before Bedtime**.
   Better yet, consider 10 hours before bedtime which has recently been suggested by new research. Caffeine disturbs sleep, even in people who do not subjectively encounter such an effect. Individuals with insomnia are often more sensitive to mild stimulants than are healthy sleepers. Caffeine is

found in items such as coffee, tea, soda, chocolate, and many over-the-counter medications (e. g., Excedrin).

5. Quit Nicotine before Bedtime.

Although some smokers maintain that smoking helps them relax, nicotine is a stimulant. Thus, smoking, dipping, or chewing tobacco should be avoided near bedtime and during the night.

6. Avoid Alcohol after Dinner.

A modest amount of alcohol often promotes the onset of sleep, but as alcohol is metabolized, sleep becomes troubled and broken. Thus, alcohol is a miserable sleep aid.

7. Sleep Medications Are Effective Only Temporarily.

Scientists have shown that sleep drugs lose their efficiency in about two to four weeks when taken regularly. Despite advertisements to the contrary, over-the-counter sleeping aids have little impact on sleep beyond the placebo effect. Over time, sleeping pills actually can make sleep problems worse. When sleeping medications have been used for a long period, withdrawal from the medication can lead to an insomnia rebound. Thus, many individuals incorrectly conclude that they "need" sleeping pills in order to sleep normally.

8. Refrain or Stay Away from Energetic Exercise Within 2 Hours of Bedtime.

Regular exercise in the late afternoon or early evening seems to aid sleep, although the helpful effect often takes several weeks to become noticeable. Exercising sporadically is not likely to improve sleep, and exercise within two hours of bedtime may elevate nervous system activity and interfere with sleep onset. Spending 20 minutes in a tub of hot water an hour or two prior to bedtime may also promote sleep.

9. Avoid Daytime Napping

Many individuals with insomnia "pay" for daytime naps with more sleeplessness at night. Thus, it is best to refrain or stay away from daytime napping. If you do nap, be sure to organize naps before 3:00 p.m.

10. A Little Snack at Bedtime May Promote Sleep.

A small bedtime snack, such a glass of warm milk, cheese, or a bowl of cereal, can help sleep. You should refrain or stay away from the following foods at bedtime: any caffeinated foods (e.g., chocolate), peanuts, beans, most raw fruits and vegetables (because they may cause gas), and high-fat foods such as potato or corn chips. Avoid snacks in the middle of the night because awakening may become affiliated with hunger.

11. Refrain or Stay Away from Excessive Liquids in the Evening.

Reducing your liquid intake will lessen the need for nighttime trips to the bathroom.

12. Do Not Try to Fall Asleep.

If you are unable to fall sleep within a prudent time (15-20 minutes) or when you notice that you are beginning to worry about falling asleep, get out of bed. Leave the bedroom and engage in a quiet action such as reading. Return to bed only when you are sleepy.

13. Don't Have Worry Time in Bed.

Lay out time earlier in the evening to review the day, plan the next day, or deal with any problems. Worrying in bed can interfere with sleep onset and cause you to have a hollow sleep.

Take One Step at a Time

It is important that you be patient with your sleep program. If you implement some of these methods, the promise of a better sleep tonight and better memory tomorrow will be realized. However, for those of you who have developed negative sleep habits over time, you will need to stick with the program and stay the course to get significant and long-lasting benefits. Habits of all kinds, including sleep habits, require repetition and practice to develop and become natural.

Conclusion

With the help of the sleep techniques and methods mentioned in this book, you will be able to solve many of the barriers that are preventing a good and healthy night's sleep. It is likely that at times you will be required to combine two or three or more of the techniques in order to return to the good night's sleep you deserve. Be patient, stay the course, and follow the guidelines presented.

Do not hesitate to contact a sleep medicine professional if your sleep problems persist. They have been specially trained to help you overcome your sleep problems. Sometimes professional help is the best course of action. Having read over this material, you will be in an excellent position to collaborate with your health care professional. You will succeed.

Be sure to visit http://www.memory-loss-facts.com/ frequently for new information and methods to enhance your brain health, memory fitness, and sleep.

For those of you interested in improving your memory, please see our practical guide, Brain Health: Simple Steps to a Better Memory. http://www.amazon.com/BrainHealthSimpleBetterebook/dp/B00 8S9A9I8

It is my earnest hope that you will use the information that I have included in this book to improve your sleep, memory, and brain and physical health.

References

1. Breslau N, Roth T, Rosenthal L, Andreski P. Sleep disturbance and psychiatric disorders: a longitudinal epidemiological study of young adults. Biol Psychiatry 1996;39:411-8.

2. Ellenbogen, J. American Academy of Neurology's 59th Annual Meeting, Boston, April 28-May 5, 2007. News release, American Academy of Neurology.

3. Edinger J, Carney CE. Overcoming Insomnia: A Cognitive-Behavioral Therapy Approach Therapist Guide. New York: Oxford University Press, 2008.

4. Pilcher, J.J.; Michalowski, K.R.; Carrigan, R.D. (2001). "The prevalence of daytime napping and its relationship to nighttime sleep". Behavioral Medicine 27 (2): 71–6.

5. Charles A. Czeisler MD, PhD (1999). "Human Biological Clock Set Back an Hour". Retrieved 2012-11-17. "The variation between our subjects, with a 95 percent level of confidence, was no more than plus or minus 16 minutes, a remarkably small range."

6. Fenn, K. M., & Hambrick, D. Z. (2011, September 12). Individual Differences in Working Memory Capacity Predict Sleep-Dependent Memory Consolidation. Journal of Experimental Psychology: General. Advance online publication. doi: 10.1037/a0025268

7. Payne, J.D. & Kensinger, E.A (2010). Sleep's role in the consolidation of emotional episodic memories. Current Directions in Psychological Science, 19(5), 290-295

8. Morin CM, Culbert JP, Schwartz SM. Nonpharmacological interventions for insomnia: a meta-analysis of treatment efficacy. Am J Psychiatry 1994;151:1172-80.

9. Chaput, J. & Tremblay, A. Adequate sleep to improve the treatment of obesity. Canadian Medical Association Journal, June 12, 2012 184:1039-1044

10. Bruno, R. M. Presentation, American Heart Association High Blood Pressure Research meeting, Washington, D.C. Sept. 21, 2012

11. Jankovic J (April 2008). "Parkinson's disease: clinical features and diagnosis". J. Neurol. Neurosurg. Psychiatr. 79 (4): 368–76. doi:10.1136/jnnp.2007.

12. Sharma, S. & Kavuru, M. (2010), sleep and metabolism: An overview. International Journal of Endocrinology Volume 2010 (2010), Article ID 270832, 12 pages doi:10.1155/2010/270832

13. Hall, M., Vasko, R., Buysse, D., Ombao, H., Qingxia, C., Cashmere, J. D., Kunpfer, D., & Thayer, J. F. Acute stress affects heart rate variability during sleep. Psychosomatic Medicine January 1, 2004 vol. 66 no. 1 56-62

14. Perlis M, Smith L.J., Lyness JM et al. Insomnia as a risk factor for onset of depression in the elderly. Behavioral Sleep Medicine 2006;4:104-13.

15. Livingston G, Watkin V, Milne B, Manela MV, Katona C. Who becomes depressed? The Islington community study of older people. J Affect Disord 2000;58:125-33.

16. Wright, J. H. & Basco, M. R. (2001) Getting your life back: The complete guide to recovery from depression. New York: Free Press

17. Ohayon, M. N. (2002). Epidemiology of insomnia: what we know and what we still need to learn. Sleep Medicine Reviews, 6(2), 97-111

18. Atkinson, J.H., Ancoli-Israel, S., Slater, M.A., Garfin, S. R., & Gillin, C. (1988). Subjective sleep disturbance in chronic pain. The Clinical Journal of Pain, 4(4):225-232

19. Phillips, B. A. & Danner, F. J. (1995). Cigarette smoking and sleep disturbance. Arch Intern Med. 1995;155(7):734-737. doi:10.1001/archinte.1995.00430070088011

20. Howell, M. J. (2011). Sleep eating. Sleep Medicine Clinics 6(4), 429-439

21. Griffin, S. J. & Trinder, J. (2007). Physical fitness, exercise, and human sleep. Psychophysiology, 15(5), 447–450

22. Herzog, N., Jauch-Chara, K., Oltmanns, K.M., & Benedict, C. (2012). Compromised sleep increases food intake in humans: two sexes, same response? Am J Clin Nutr, 95(2) 531; doi:10.3945/ajcn.111.028647

23. Ullrich, P. M., M.A. & Lutgendorf, S.K. (2002). Journaling About Stressful Events: Effects of Cognitive Processing and Emotional Expression. Annals of Behavioral Medicine, 24(3)

24. Krakow, B.,Hollifield,M., Johnston,L., Koss, M., Schrader, R., Warner, T.D.,Tandberg, D.,Lauriello, J.,McBride,L., Cutchen, L.,Cheng,D. Emmons,S. Germain, A.,Melendrez, D.,Sandoval, D.,& Prince, H. (2001). Imagery rehearsal therapy for chronic

nightmares in sexual assault survivors with posttraumatic stress disorder. JAMA. 2001;286(5):537-545. doi:10.1001/jama.286.5.537

Resources

American Academy of Sleep Medicine: http://www.aasmnet.org/

American Sleep Association: www.sleepassociation.org

Center for Disease Control: www.cdc.gov

Food and Drug Administration: www.fda.gov

National Institutes of Health (NIH): www.nih.gov

National Sleep Foundation: www.sleepfoundation.org

Restless Leg Syndrome (RLS) Foundation: http://www.rls.org/

World Health Organization: www.who.int

Thank You

Thank you for reading Good Sleep for Brain Health: Sleep Better Tonight for a Better Memory Tomorrow. When you are done reading the book, please take a few minutes to write a review where you purchased it. This is a way for me to improve future editions and, of course, my writing style. Also, if you found it helpful, please tell your friends and send them to the site where you purchased it.

Best,

Dr. M. Chris Wolf

www.ingramcontent.com/pod-product-compliance
Lightning Source LLC
Chambersburg PA
CBHW070540290526
45790CB00002B/579